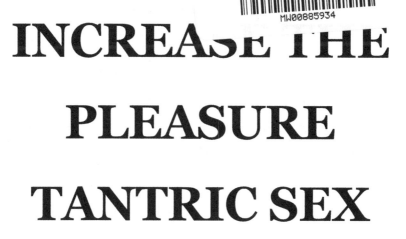

INCREASE THE

PLEASURE

TANTRIC SEX

Give Your Partner the Best Sex Experience Using Sex Positions Based on Modern Sex Life.Use Yoga and Meditation Essentials to Overcome Anxiety and Increase Intimacy

By

Barbara Moore

The information in the following pages is broadly considered a truthful and accurate account of facts and as such, any inattention, use, or misuse of the information in question by the reader will render any resulting actions solely under their purview. There are no scenarios in which the publisher or the original author of this work can be in any fashion deemed liable for any hardship or damages that may befall them after undertaking information described herein.

Additionally, the information in the following pages is intended only for informational purposes and should thus be thought of as universal. As befitting its nature, it is presented without assurance regarding its prolonged validity or interim quality. Trademarks that are mentioned are done without written consent and can in no way be considered an endorsement from the trademark holder.

Table of Content

Introduction

Though the origin of Tantra is a bit tricky to pin down, it's pretty well-accepted by most that it found its start in ancient Indian spiritual practice around about 5,000 years ago. Despite its start in the eastern world, tantra and navatantric sex is a global concept practiced today by millions. Tantra and tantric sex techniques to fit the modern world are always being expanded and traversed in order to discover new ways of maintaining the most intimate connections between partners. Tantric sex has very little to do with reaching a sexual peak, and everything to do with building a deep emotional connection. Whether or not you experience orgasm is irrelevant.

The sexual connection, in this case, is the journey, not the destination. You'll find among these lessons, many benefits that come with practicing tantric sex, but in the case of the experience being all about the journey, tantric sex can work very well as an all-natural promotion of sexual virility, and a solution to low sexual libido. Tantric sex asks the individual to become familiar and comfortable with their own sexual being, and then to experience pleasure sharing this experience with another. These practices seek to worship the bodies and deliver intense pleasure to one another through their application.

Tantra is nowhere near only about sex. Practicing tantric sex and tantric living means embracing a concentration on one's own breath, thoughts, and alignment with the ultimate self. Truly, only after aligning with your own self, can you achieve ultimate alignment with another. A tantric master is acutely attentive to his or her own physical movements, both within the external world and within one's own internal body.

Our understanding of tantric sex, and tantra as a philosophy and way of life, in general, has been warped, skewed, and watered down so that most of us are left with the layman's understanding that tantric sex is about wild, tawdry, love-making. That's not to say it can't be, but it isn't necessarily. First and foremost, tantra was a spiritual practice and a habit of breathing. The tantric observance is also about exploring other intimate parts of the relationship that are not just sex. It's about finding intimate pleasure in those places.

Tantra is a commitment of thoughts, beliefs, behaviors, and the awareness of these when interacting with others, both platonically and sexually. If your connection with your partner is suffering from a weak signal, the implementation of tantric sex, alone or together, can transform and reignite the intimate and sexual experiences you have with your partner. With a tantric perspective, the experience becomes about identifying pleasures and desires and giving them proper recognition. Then, using that power for leverage in experiencing extreme indulgence in those desires. This can definitely be achieved on your own, and probably should be, before sharing the experience with another. In many practices of tantric sex, there is no contact with genitals at all, but the same, and better, enhancement of the sexual experience comes to fruition. Instead of reaching climax, the goal is to see how much pleasure you can experience and where you can follow your own sexual energy, and then the sexual energy created between you and another.

Until now, perhaps you've struggled with a truly intimate connection with someone. Perhaps the sexual connection that you once had has become dull and stagnant. If you've only fantasized about rekindling your own sexual power and deep sexual chemistry, you're done searching. Tantric sex will deliver these to you. When you experience alignment and union with yourself, there is a distinct and enlightened satisfaction. But as you grow and expand that understanding of yourself, this can be explored together with your partner in a very spiritually fulfilling way that will bring your union into a tighter link, undoubtedly.

Tantric sex is a way to bring two individuals together to congregate in each other's being fully, dually. Then, taking that energy into dissolving that duality and becoming one being experiencing ultimate pleasure. BY embracing this new way of experience together, partners stand by each other in support and help each other to reach new heights of enlightenment. Whether with yourself or with another, it's common to experience a lack of sexual awareness and pleasure.

Our lives are so dictated by the routine that we cannot help but start to apply that way of thinking and behaving in other parts of our lives. Our brains do this in order to organize and protect us or mitigate damage, but after a while, it becomes evident that these practices once put in place are actually now the problem and not the solution. We become largely driven by the routine rather than the inspiration.

Tantric sex will take you from the hum-drum automatic routine to a deeply satisfying gift to yourself, and perhaps others. If you're reading this, your alarm is going off, and it's time to answer the bell and wake up your body and your ultimate self. When practicing with another, tantric sex especially focuses on the giving of pleasure to the other, rather than the taking of it for oneself. We are worshipping each other's bodies and want to show the utmost service and gratitude by delivering pleasure in the most powerful ways we know how.

These ways may have eluded you before, but not now. You are on the journey to self-discovery and liberation. The ego takes a back seat as you seek to satisfy your partner. You want to deliver the ultimate experience for them. Connect with them in all the ways you can. This is tantra. Think about love. Act with love. Touch with love. Practice patience and compassion, and you're easily on your way to awakening your senses together. At the roots of a tantric bond with another is a relationship that honors the spiritual being, the body, the mind, the heart, and the soul. You will both be very present at the moment, oblivious to the rest of the world, sharing energy.

Chapter 1: Tantra

So, what is tantric sex at its core? It's pretty in-depth, and here, we'll talk all about what tantric sex is, the concepts behind it, and why it matters.

Tantric Sex at the Core

Tantric sex is a type of sexual experience that involves more of slowing down, enjoying what you're doing, and feeling the fun and experience of the moment. It's not quick sex, but more slow, methodical, and fun to experience.

The idea behind it is that it's the opposite of a quickie, rushed sex, or anything that seems almost quick and meaningless. This is all about enjoying the other person, and in general, involves increasing intimacy.

The goal of it isn't to just have sex, but it's to experience a deep connection with your partner and is great for serious couples who enjoy it.

An older Practice

This type of sex isn't just some generic type of sex that you have, but instead, it's a methodical, older process that's important to do. It's an ancient Hindu activity that's been occurring for at least five millennia. So yes, this has been around for a little bit.

The concept behind it is that it's the waving and expansion of different energies, bringing them together in a deep, intimate connection with another being.

It is very slow, and the goal of it is to create a connection between the body and mind. This connection is said to bring about powerful orgasms as a result of it.

It can be done by just about anyone who is physically able to do it. If you want to reboot your sex life, or even find a deeper meaning into the act of making love, this is how you do it.

For most people in this day and age, we all focus on just the action itself, getting it done so we can go about our business. But, does that really build a connection? Are you really focused on your partner? This is what you have to realize happens with tantric sex.

If you are looking for a good way to compare this, a quickie is literally like a takeout food, whereas tantric sex is a five-star meal that you eat in the restraint. With this type of sex, you're not spending as much time just getting it done just to get it done, but it's slow, savoring, and wonderful to experience, and in turn, is a delicious and mesmerizing experience.

This can also bring some space back into your love life. Do you sometimes think you're just having sex just to have sex? Do you sometimes feel like you're not really engaged in the act of sex? Well, that's the problem. For most people, sex is just a quick and dirty thing, rather than an intimate, wholesome action between two parties. That in turn, will cause your relationship to feel hollow, boring, and not worth it.

But, with tantric sex, you can change the way it all feels. Instead of just taking things like activity and not really putting more emphasis on it than that, tantric sex involves the action of sex, the doingness of it, but also the connection shared between you and the other being you're with.

It's deeper, more thoughtful for both parties, and a ton of fun.

Why Try Tantric sex?

There is a reasoning behind trying tantric sex. Tantric sex for one, ash been around for thousands of years. It must work pretty well if you're looking to do something different, and have a deeper, more thoughtful connection with another person.

But, if you want to extend the effort and time into sex, you'll start to get a much more intense ecstasy from it.

16

Which means a much more intense orgasm.

It does work, and there are even celebrities that will do his with their partners, and it's part of the reason why some people will stay together with one another.

And sometimes, it builds that deep, intimate connection with that person that you want. If you feel like your relationship with your partner is a little stale and boring, this is one of the easiest always to spice things up.

If you're sick of doing the same old, same old in bed, then tantric sex is for you. If you want to become more intimate with the person you love, this is for you. If you would like to reconnect with the one that you love, especially after raising kids, or a stressful day, this is for you.

In the hustle and bustle of our world, we might not think that we have time for this type of sex, but it's a great form of sex, and it can change your life and the lives of others too.

The concept behind this is where you start to realize that all experience that you have, including sexual intercourse, is a personal thing, and has the potential to transform your ability to understand yourself. Everything in life does this, not just having sex, but we're going to talk about the sexual aspects of this in there.

The idea behind this as well is to be aware and enlightened. You're more aware when you're experiencing tantric sex than you would be if you're just having a quickie with your partner. Perhaps you haven't really looked at your partner all that much recently, or maybe you haven't really thought about anything besides everything you want to do after sex.

Well, tantric sex lets you achieve that awareness of the other person, and it's pretty interesting.

While it does have roots in ancient tantra, it's wonderful for those who want to experience a deeper and more immersive sexual experience.

And what's more, is that tantric sex doesn't involve being spiritual at all. You don't have to be a Hindu to participate in tantric sex, but you can apply these principles in order to have a better life and learn about it as well.

Everything you do during tantric sex is a connection. Whether you both synchronize your breathing together, look a one another, or even touch one another while having intercourse. Unlike other types of sex, it isn't a quick and dirty activity, but instead helps prolong the experience with your partner, and deepen the connection with one another.

So now that you know at the core what tantric sex is, let's discuss the beliefs and the benefits of tantric sex.

The Benefits of Tantric Sex

Tantric sex has a myriad of different benefits, and here, we'll highlight and discuss in detail some of the benefits tantric sex has to offer.

Rejuvenates your Sexual Health

Tantric sex is wonderful for sexual health, especially for women, but men do as well.

When you have a lot of orgasms frequently in your brain, it stimulates brain waves, and the chemistry that you have will alter as well.

For many people, sex is used as a way to relax, but it's more than just a simple ejaculation or climax. It's a way to help release those energies which are tied up.

Think about your current sexual health. Do you orgasm a lot? Do you sometimes have sex without being fully aroused, or even an orgasm? Sometimes this happens, especially with women. Some women take much longer to get aroused or even to experience orgasms, which means that for them, sex is more than an activity they do to benefit their partner rather than themselves.

But, when you use tantric sex, the idea is to benefit both parties, not just the guy who is having sex, but the woman as well. That means you'll both have amazing orgasms, and you'll feel better about sex as well. You'll want to have sex more, and sex will be better, more meaningful for you.

That can do a number of great things on both your physical and mental health, and we'll discuss that here.

Depression and Stress Relief

Depression and stress are two of the biggest mental hurdles that we have in our world today. However, sex is a way to help relieve it. But, if you're just having quickie after quickie, without really having a deeper, more immersive connection with your partner, can you really say that it's stress-relieving?

Chances are, it's not. You need to have that long, relaxing sexual experience to be happier. While five hours might be excessive, for some people, that's significantly more than the five minutes they were having beforehand.

Tantric sex helps with stress and depression, and it can help you feel better too. When you orgasm, a lot of the stress you experience while having sex will magically melt away, resulting in you being happier and much healthier too.

It can even affect the brain chemistry too, probably in ways you've already experienced, but they're worth mentioning regardless, for example, the endocrine glands start to increase, meaning a much higher high, some serotonin excreted, some DHEA, and testosterone too, which will affect your physical wellness too. All of this is there, and there are even some studies that say when you have more orgasms, you'll experience greater mental health and wellness.

Sex isn't just a temporary orgasm and temporary happiness, either. With tantric sex, it takes it to the next level, ups the ante a little bit. When you experience tantric sex, you're experiencing a more intimate and personal connection with the person you love, and that in turn, can make you feel utterly amazing.

Tantric sex is a good thing to have, and it's something that, with the way things are sometimes, can really help you mentally feel good.

Depends on the Bond

How many times do you have sex with your partner, and it feels almost...forgettable? Sex shouldn't be some forgettable experience. Some of us have sex for the sake of our partners, and sometimes, we just have sex in order to have sex.

But, with tantric sex, it changes the game. With tantric sex, you're using that connection you've got with the other person, and in turn, building more understanding with the other person, and some wellness and happiness too. You will feel more in-tune with your partner, and much happier as well you'll feel the connection grow between the two of you.

And it isn't just a physical connection, and it's a mental connection too. If you sometimes feel the distance between you and your partner, having tantric sex will help you with enjoying the moment, enjoying your partner, and making things better between the two of you as well. So yes, it will help develop a healthier connection and a deeper understanding.

Physical benefits

Orgasms do possess a physical benefit too. They can improve your health a lot, and it can help with making your body stronger too through cardiovascular health, endocrine, and immune function, along with nervous system health too. If you have tantric sex at least twice a week, it releases an antibody that's called immunoglobulin A, or also called IgA, which protects your body from illness.

Orgasms also can help alleviate depression and help you feel and look younger. Some also believe it'll make your lifespan stronger, strengthening your immune system, and improving the overall health of you too. However, there are still studies that need to be done to verify these results completely.

But, sexual experience and exposure to semen do help boost the moods I most women, and in many cases, it can help with your mood enhancements, your emotional bands, and ultimate intimacy too.

Men and women both can benefit from this too. This isn't just one or the other, but having sex together will provide these benefits since it'll be an activity both of you participate in too.

There is also the fact that it can be a wonderful cardio for the body. Sex burns a lot of calories, and orgasm does too. That's why it's imperative you consider this since even making love requires energy, and if you're going for a long time, it can be a wonderful workout.

It also naturally relaxes the body. Tantric sex, in particular, does it, since you're calming both the body and the mind down in order to be in-sync with your partner. That mutual togetherness alone stimulates your vagus nerve, thereby relaxing the body and promoting wellness too. Over time, you'll start to feel the muscles that were stretched start to relax, and you'll practice diaphragmic breathing too.

Tantric sex is great for the physical body, and it is a good thing to do for you, not just because it feels great, but because it makes you feel great too.

A Woman's Orgasm

Tantric sex, in particular, will help with a woman's orgasm. There is a big difference between the ordinary orgasm that you get from sex and tantric orgasms, and oftentimes, it will change how the woman feels.

Many times, these can last for hours, and in women, this can change their sexual health. There is a command during a tantric orgasm that reaches your brains' control center and hat's through the hypothalamus and the pituitary gland, and I will majorly benefit the sex life of women in particular.

A lot of the hormone oxytocin gets released during a tantric orgasm, and this alone can boost your mood, the position you feel in life, your passion, your emotion, and your social skills. Having tantric sex can do all of this, and I can benefit you in your daily activities.

It'll Make You More Patient

Tantric sex isn't just for sexual pleasure, and it helps with developing life skills and building on weaknesses.

Do you sometimes kind of just want to get it done rather than go through the deep connection w=in the moment? You might not even realize it because hormones fuel your body and mind, but tantric sex promotes patience, which is something of a virtue that everyone can have during sex. However, this can also help you to build a deeper, better connection with your partner.

Sometimes, tantric sex is a little bit awkward, since many people aren't used to just sitting there, focusing on their partner, breathing together, and developing a real look at the person they're with. Some people don' even realize they do this either.

Do you tend to have sex with either your eyes closed or the lights off? While dimming the lights aids to the ambiance, tantric sex makes it a little different. Tantric sex is actually a meditative process, and they encourage you to hold back the orgasm. It didn't denial, and it's your conscious effort to hold it back so you and your partner can have a conscious moment together.

Patience develops naturally from this. You might not even realize it, but you learn to understand and appreciate your partner a whole lot more after engaging in tantric sex.

Those things that used to piss you off every now and then? Well, now, if you practice tantric sex, this patience develops, and you grow stranger with your partner over time.

Helps with Problem Solving

This might seem a bit strange, but for those starting, it's a different type of activity that you might not be used to. Those who are beginners or new to the experience might realize that the positions required for tantric sex are much more varied than just the same old positions.

Some of them might not even provide much pleasure to you either.

This requires you to work together with your partner. It has sex a team activity, where both of you need to talk it out and work together as well, in order to enjoy pleasure.

This can oftentimes be embarrassing because both of you are vulnerable in this state, but it helps with problem-solving skills and builds that connection. Plus, if you're a team, you'll have a much stronger connection outside of the bedroom, and work to solve the problems you have going on outside of the bedroom as well.

This also stimulates creativity. That's because we're embracing the concept of "supra sexuality," which expresses our purpose, which is creativity and empowerment in order to unlock our full potential. Sex might be used to create human life, of course, but it also brings forth new and creative actions that will help you experience a pleasurable sensation in order to achieve the goals that you have during intercourse as well.

Let's You Be Selfless

Do you sometimes feel like your partner is a little selfish in the bedroom? Do you sometimes feel you might be a tiny bit selfish? It might be because of the fact that you're not withholding your orgasm.

There is a benefit to doing this, and that's something to mention. Oftentimes, people don't realize that tantric sex offers the power of liberation, which allows for you to have an amazing experience that is often compared to glimpsing into the cosmic consciousness of the other person, fostering a deeper, more responsible understanding of the person.

Oftentimes, some people don't realize how selfish they are until they have the tantric orgasm, which will change their life and blow their minds. Oftentimes, they might not even realize that they are like this until it happens.

But for the other person, it can benefit them too. Sex is a two-person activity, and if you and your partner are both not talking out what will benefit the other person, and your partner isn't a little bit selfless, it can cause problems later on. You need to walk into this with the idea of supporting one another into orgasms, since this will help others remember and get a better idea of giving, rather than just receiving.

We're a culture focused on the receiving end of sex. While it's fun, also giving to the other person can have some marked benefit to you as well.

Chapter 2: Pleasure

This might be the reason why you're practicing tantric sex period. If it is then great, and here, we'll discuss the tantric orgasm in its entirety. It's a little more in-depth than you'd think it is, and it's something that can change your life for the better. We'll highlight the perks and the different parts of the tantric orgasm, and how with this act, it can change you for the better.

What Is It?

When we talk about the orgasm, it's usually a taboo thing. Mentioning orgasms at the dinner table or with family is something that, unless you live in an open household, is something you either don't do, or you can't. There's a lot about orgasms that we don't discuss, simply because of the taboo nature of it. But, did you know that your sexual health, mental health, and your physical health can be affected by your orgasms?

Many people don't realize that not all types of orgasms are equal, and one of the most powerful ones is the tantric orgasm. That's because it allows you to achieve everything that you desire and help to undo all of the harm that manifests in your life, helping you get what you really want out of it.

The tantric orgasm takes your orgasm to the next level and is oftentimes called the full-body orgasm. We'll discuss some of the different orgasms to really help highlight the tantric orgasm.

Types of Orgasms

You can have an orgasm that isn't just sexual. An orgasm is the sudden release of energy that's not sexual all the time in nature, but some orgasms do happen through sex.

A sexual orgasm is an orgasm that happens through the art of sex, and usually, it's the peak of your sexual energy. However, it can be on a different level too.

There is also the energy orgasm, which might be the sudden release of energy that's accumulated. Did you know that a seizure is a type of orgasm since it's the release of energies? Yawning is too, so you can actually suddenly release a bunch of energy, and many times, this is a sudden, uncontrolled release.

Have you ever felt a sudden burst of energy and then suddenly felt the low come back after a little bit? That's the effects of an orgasm in place since this is usually the sudden release of energy and then the sudden realization.

You can control your orgasms as well, and you can control this sudden energy as well.

Tantric sex is kind of the full-body orgasm that you can enjoy. It's the sudden blow-up, the explosion, and the release.

But the tantric orgasm is a full-on orgasm that frees up the body, and oftentimes it will re-sensitize the body when people are experiencing it. It's literally an orgasm that's so powerful you can't really hold it back.

The Valley Orgasm

The valley orgasm is usually what we call the genital orgasm because it's mostly just around that arousal, where we feel the savoring flavor, the sudden rise, and then the fall and then back to normal. It's a much-cantered form of orgasm, and oftentimes, once you expand it, the sensation can then go through the full-body, allowing you to feel that nourished and exhausted wave as you go along.

Full body, in contrast, is usually when you feel it throughout the whole body experience the power of the orgasm. Many times, people think this is just the whole body screaming, but it actually can make the sudden sensation of the orgasm flow away from the genitalia, penetrating your entire body.

It isn't always the screaming and writhing, it's the feeling of the sudden release of the energy, and it can affect how you feel afterward.

Orgasming without an Ejaculation

The crazy thing about this is that it can cause men to orgasm without ejaculation. It's actually not very difficult, and the main reason why some men can do this is that the focus is off the genitalia, and it's more on the entire body, and you feel the full-on intensity, and from there, the sensation of the orgasm starts to spread through the body.

Why should you try to go for this type of orgasm? Well, we'll highlight the different kinds of physical and mental benefits that come about as a result of a tantric orgasm.

The Benefits of Tantric Orgasms

Tantric orgasms are different because they offer more than just a mere genitalia orgasm. Orgasms, however, do lead to a feeling of both euphoria and pleasure, which reduce your depression, stress, and anxiety levels, and help to boost your immune system too naturally.

Plus, tantric orgasms allow for you to burn a lot of calories, relax, and also release those tension points in the body, not just from the genitalia. If your sleep quality is suffering, you can always have an orgasm, and it will help with this. It also increases circulation within the brain and the body, leading to a sharper brain, and better mental clarity. It also alleviates pain, regenerates cells, and also reduces aging in the body too.

Orgasms also release oxytocin in the body, which allows you to have stronger feelings of intimacy. A tantric orgasm focuses on releasing a lot of this, improving the bond between you and your partner, and making the connection between both of out even stronger.

But, it's more than just a physical benefit, it also will help you in a spiritual sense as well. The big thing about an orgasm is, after it happens, your body opens up to a state where you're very receptive. All of the parts of the body start to feel the flow of energies, and a tantric orgasm does this to the whole body, not just to the genitalia. It can align you in a spiritual and physical sense and allow you to increase the vibration of your physical and mental perspectives too, so it helps with blending each aspect of yourself into different ways. During orgasms, the awareness of your ego dissolves, so you attain a state of infinite nature, and that's why sex and orgasms are spiritual tools. Orgasms are one of the best ways to attain enlightenment, and that's why tantric sex is so powerful. You become more vulnerable and excited, and you also feel a much higher sense of awareness, and this sexual practice can and will change you.

You can even manifest what you want in life through an orgasm. It isn't just the conception of children through sex, but it can be pretty much anything. What many don't know is that the tantric orgasm allows you to manifest everything that you can possibly want in life through the practice of an orgasm. This will enable you to focus on and experience the moment of your orgasm fully, and when you focus on this at such a deep, intimate level, you conceive everything that you want.

Remember that, when you do have an orgasm all of that energy that's been building up is then released, and you can practically shoot out all of that energy that you want and desire, causing a manifestation of whatever it is that you want into the reality of the moment, making it possible to pretty much-attaining everything that you can possibly achieve just through an orgasm.

Sounds a little crazy, right? Well, you should understand that this is a process, and you want to manifest experience through this orgasm, and it can help release the negative thoughts. You should definitely consider this form of orgasm to be one of the most powerful.

How Many Times Should You Experience a Tantric Orgasm?

Well, that depends on how much you need it. Some people need to look at the energy that's there. Look at orgasms as a form of relieving the tension and reaching a higher state, and not just using them for an escape.

Some people do use these solely to escape the harshness of our world, but that won't help you. That's not a healthy use of the orgasm, but if you do it in a way where it's healthy for you to do, and for you to possess, then you'll be much better off.

So, some people can have a tantric orgasm once a week. Some people, if they really need to align their spiritual energies, they might do it more often than anything else. The big thing to remember here- you have to do this for yourself, for what you want out of a tantric orgasm, and for your own personal benefit. Don't worry so much about how you do it, but instead focus on the process of doing it.

Edging and how It Builds the Tantric Orgasm

One way to bring about the tantric orgasm and the experience is to delay the orgasm. This is a way to push yourself into a higher rate of arousal, helping you experience the deeper, more forceful orgasms that can help you feel better, and reach towards the full body.

Delaying orgasms helps you feel the power of an orgasm, and it can be more than just a sexual orgasm in many cases, but a physical manifestation as well.

Edging is the best way to do it, and you can do this to yourself or your partner. For men, it is said to bring about

35

very powerful orgasms, but it works pretty well for women too.

It is a way where you get yourself to the point of orgasm and then stopping, and then doing this again and again. It feels amazing, and it helps you achieve orgasm, and is a big part of tantric sex.

One way I like to do this is to try it on your partner, and from there, do it on yourself. Your ca docs this, stop, and then switch it up, taking turns bringing one another to climax, sliding back down, and then doing this again, and finally reaching the finale after a bit. It's a good way to experience this type of orgasm, especially if you're someone who is used to always having quick orgasms. It's a good way to stimulate the body too, and it can be a lot of fun.

This state that you get into isn't always just from your genitals, though. The idea behind it is to feel the orgasmic state within your body. This is definitely a different feeling. An orgasm is a burst of energy flowing through the body, and you should understand that the orgasm doesn't always have ejaculation at the end of this.

The idea of it is to feel it in your entire body and let go of the idea that you have always just to feel it in your genitals. This pulls you into a deep, orgasmic state. It may not mean that you even have a writhing or any destabilizing with the sensation. The idea behind it is to feel the energies that come in, and the union of everything that's going on in your life. It's a way to be subtle with the way your energies are, and you'll know the orgasmic state. It's a burst of energy, but it doesn't always have to be a violent or very apparent thing.

It can be subtle and understanding that will help you awaken the orgasmic state within your body. It will allow you to experience exactly what you want out of tantra, allowing you to desensitize the body completely.

Sometimes the best way to figure out what you like from a tantric orgasm is to figure out what you like from your own body, and what type of energies you want to release from this, and some of the different faces of that. This can be a deep, lifelong journey that you may not realize you've got to embark on to understand truly, but understanding the different nuances of your body will change you, and you'll realize that there is a deeper, more effective form of orgasm that you will experience, that you will love. Tantric orgasms can change your life, and it's a way to look at the energy from orgasm in a completely different way, and in a way that'll allow you to fully understand and get a good grasp on what you need to do to experience the lifelong effects of this amazing feeling.

The key differences between tantric sex, and what you're Having Now

Tantric sex and our regular "sexual" sex is very different, and in some ways, people don't even realize the impact of tantric sex, and how it can change the way you have sex.

We'll highlight the key differences and why tantric sex should be the focus for couples looking to have a spicier, better sex life than ever before.

A different pathway

Regular sex has three different stages: foreplay, the act of intercourse, and of course, the climax or ending. Once that's done, it actually is the end, and usually, you're done. Sometimes you have sex, and you go back to your normal life.

But tantric sex is different. Tantric sex has zero linear progression. You might not even have an orgasm until after foreplay and intercourse, or maybe even just foreplay brings you to that level. The idea behind it isn't to just focus on the orgasm, and don't use the orgasm as the ending point. It takes away that idea and makes it so that you're not as hung up on it.

The energies that are there

The energy that's in a regular bout of sex is different. It's purely sexual, penis or vagina against another genitalia, and the whole act is physical. Whether it be kissing, rubbing, pinching, or even penetration, the idea behind it is physical, and not as mental. Oftentimes, people might not even look at one another, and it is something that you need to realize makes tantric sex a little different.

The connection that's there during tantric sex isn't just a physical manifestation, but it's also a different type of manifestation of energy. This is more than just sexual energy, but they try to expand that energy from the genitalia out to the rest of the body so that it can cause pleasure in different forms. The pleasure and energies that are there are actually not just the actions of the movements of the body, but the way your partner feels, and the mental energy that's there. It allows you to have a deeper feeling with this, and it is a much more intimate activity tan just regular sex in most cases.

Working together

The thing with regular sex is, usually the endgame of it is an orgasm, to have that release, and then you're done. You're more focused on that than just working and experiencing the moment together.

The crazy thing about tantric sex is you can have an orgasm not just from the act of intercourse alone. Some people have an orgasm from massages, from light foreplay, even pinching or biting the nipples can result in a tantric orgasm. The idea of it is to stop worrying so much about orgasms, and instead, focus on the moment.

You want to make sure that your breathing is similar to your partner's, and it isn't out of sorts, and it isn't labored or wavering. You also want to keep eye contact with one another.

This is something that most people don't realize they don't do when they engage in regular sex. Whether it be doggy-style or even just turning the lights off instead of on, people are scared to look at one another. Maybe it's the vulnerability of the moment, but it actually can change the way it makes you feel. Tantric sex brings you out of the "only me" mindset during sex, making you more selfless, and helping you attain that connection over time.

Time Spent

The time spent during sex usually varies, but most people usually don't spend more than an hour together in the bedroom, unless, of course, they want to go long. Sometimes, the quickie sessions last all but five minutes, and that's it. But, here's the thing, tantric sex can last a long time, several hours at that.

That's partial because they aren't trying to do this just to get off, but instead, they want to submerge into a way where they can cyclically go together and experience intercourse. The crazy thing about this is that tantric sex causes more orgasms and more powerful orgasms than standard sex does.

The end of the game isn't a depletion of the physical energies, but instead, you're both experiencing a cyclical direction of you both experiencing the fun and pleasure of one another, and the pleasure and intensity spent.

Chapter 3: Chakras

Yin and Yang

Everybody perceives the image: the little high contrast half circles that twirl into one another, with a spot of the contrary shading on either side. Just by taking a gander at it, its most fundamental significance is clear: look after equalization. In any case, the importance of Yin and Yang goes a lot further than that.

Foundation

Scarcely any old ways of thinking have been as powerful as Taoism. Created in the fourth century B.C., the way of thinking is revolved around the accomplishment of 'the Way' and discovering agreement and parity inside. At the core of this way of thinking is the image that has come to speak to it as its most identifiable angle: the Yin and Yang.

The Image

Considerably more than simply the tattoo on the person from your hand to hand fighting class, the Yin Yang conveys with it a profound implying that is as basic as it is significant. To get it, how about we separate the image into its two constituent parts. The Yin, or the clouded side, is related with everything hard, negative, cool, wet, and ladylike. The Yang, or the light side, is related to things delicate, positive, warm, dry, and manly.

In any case, in spite of the brutal juxtaposition of their appearances, Yin and Yang are not direct inverses. Truth be told, it is significant that each side has a smidgen of the other in it. That is the way you end up with a wave's peak being Yang and its trough being Yin.

Yin and Yang in Regular Day to Day Existence

Actually, Yin and Yang are in all things, and most things are a smidgen of both. An eggshell is Yang. However, the egg inside is Yin. Wheat in the field is Yang, yet once it is collected, it moves toward becoming Yin. One can transform into the other, and the best things in life lie at the juncture of the two.

The idea of Yin and Yang is at the core of Chinese drug. Have you at any point pondered, for instance, why Chinese individuals drink so much boiling water? It is tied in with offsetting the body's Yin and Yang. It couldn't be any more obvious, the equalization of the two is the most significant angle. The two powers are restricting however integral.

Nourishment

Chinese nourishment, likewise, is fragmented without a comprehension of Yin and Yang. Yang sustenances are those who are fiery or sweet. Like the glow that Yang instills, Yang sustenances are frequently those in warm hues like red and orange. Yin sustenances are those who are salty or harsh. They are cool in shading and are regularly developed in water. Models incorporate tofu and soy sauce.

Everybody realizes plain tofu is not the most tantalizing dish. In any case, pair it with some bean stew peppers, a la the Mapo style, and it is the most loved in Chinese cafés around the world. Despite the fact that all in all, a few dishes are more one than different, components of both Yin and Yang ought to be available inside.

The Human Body

Despite sex, Yin and Yang are both presents in the human body too, and their quality comes and goes with the time. Normally, Yang is more grounded during the day when the sun is out, and it is warm. What's more, Yin takes over during the evening, when its agent, the moon, comes to join the party.

The Impact of Yin and Yang

Furthermore, however, Taoism is more a way of thinking than a religion, it instructs that there is a higher power known to man, 'the Way.' Yet as opposed to being all great or all awful, it is a tad bit of both, much the same as Yin and Yang.

Yin Yang is maybe the most known and reported idea utilized inside Taoism.

A beginning definition: Yin/Yang: Two parts that together complete wholeness. Yin and yang are likewise the beginning stage for change. When something is entire, by definition, it is perpetual and complete. So when you split something into equal parts – yin/yang, it irritates the balance of wholeness. The two parts are pursuing each other as they look for another offset with one another.

The word Yin turns out to signify the "obscure side," and Yang is the "bright side."

Yin Yang is the idea of duality framing an entirety. We experience instances of Yin and Yang consistently. As models: night (Yin) and day (Yang), female (Yin), and male (Yang). More than a large number of years, a lot has been arranged and assembled under different Yin Yang classification frameworks.

The image for Yin Yang is known as the Taijitu. The vast majority simply consider it the yin yang image in the west. The taijitu image has been found in more than one culture, and throughout the years, has come to speak to Taoism.

Essential Concepts Defining the Nature of Yin Yang

Yin Yang is not static. The idea of Yin and Yang streams and changes with time. A straightforward model is contemplating how the day steadily streams into the night. Be that as it may, the length of day and night are evolving. As the earth ages, its turn is easing back, making the length of day and night get longer. Day and night are not static substances. Some of the time, changes in the connection between Yin and Yang can be sensational, where one viewpoint can simply change into the other.

Neither Yin nor Yang is total. Nothing is totally Yin or totally Yang. Every viewpoint contains the starting point for the other angle. For instance, the day moves toward becoming night, and after that night moves toward becoming day. Yin and Yang are reliant upon one another with the goal that the meaning of one requires the definition for the other to be finished.

The summation of Yin and Yang structure an entirety. One impact of this is: as one perspective expands different declines to keep up the general equalization of the entirety.

The parity of Yin Yang can be slanted due to outside impacts. Four potential lopsided characteristics exist abundance in Yin and Yang and lack in Yin and Yang. These irregular characteristics can be combined: so an abundance of Yin can likewise recreate a Yang lack and the other way around.

For instance, this idea is particularly significant for Chinese mending rehearses. So an abundance of Yang brings about a fever. An overabundance of Yin could mean the amassing of liquids in the body. Chinese mending looks at an individual's wellbeing by utilizing the eight standards: Internal and External improvements, Deficiency and Excesses, Cold and Heat, Yin and Yang.

Yin Yang can be subdivided into extra Yin and Yang viewpoints. For instance, a Yang part of Heat: can be additionally subdivided into a Yin warm or Yang consuming.

Extra rules that characterize Yin and Yang characteristics exist. The ideas recorded here are only a beginning stage to delineate the idea of Yin and Yang. For the most part, as a training, Taoism works superbly of not codifying life. Incidentally, this wasn't valid about yin Yang, since over history, many Taoist's have attempted to codify what is Yin and what is Yang. Commonly Taoist writings will list a couple of instances of Yin and Yang and afterward wander off to the following point. For instance, return to the Taoist entry cited above from the Tao Te Ching. You will find a couple of extra angles to Yin and Yang. However, the perusing is certainly not a total definition either. The writer of this completely anticipates that you, as the peruser, should go out and to investigate the thoughts all alone. You can endlessly dive into Yin Yang because of its relative nature.

Extra material for Yin Yang can be perused here:

The Flow of Yin and Yang

Presently overlook all that you have found out about Yin and Yang for a minute. A more clear comprehension of Yin Yang requires thinking once more into the Tao. The Tao can be considered as the crucial outright. Upon assessment: the nature of the Tao extends out. This procedure of extension characterizes an example, parting separated into better and better designs. Yin and Yang are where recognition demarks the Tao's venture into one and afterward one into two.

Taoism, as a training, appreciates inspecting designs. Throughout the years incalculable organizations of Taoism have framed and a considerable amount of writing composed over the depiction and portrayal of these examples. Frequently Taoists utilize the idea of Yin Yang as a natural beginning layout to work with examples.

For instance, Qigong depends on examples of breath and physical development. Information on real examples frames the premise of this Taoist practice to keep a body sound. The human body and its developments are separated by Yin and Yang classifications. So the chest area compares to the Yang, while the lower body roots into the Yin. The body's middle is the place the Yin and Yang meet. Qi Gong activities are assembled and clarified as far as Yin and Yang to help classify the body's harmonies into working practice. The information of Yin or Yang is not required to perform Qi Gong. Rather, it is an extra channel that causes individuals to interface with the training.

Another model is Taoist divination inside the Book of Changes/I Ching. Divination in Taoism is a routine with regards to looking at human communications dependent on surely understood mental examples. To create an outcome, either coins or yarrow stalks are hurled down to shape an example. The examples produced compare to Yin and Yang characterized characteristics. The idea of the Yin and Yang example is connected to the brain research existing apart from everything else to return guidance for the individual posing the inquiry.

Yin Yang is a key part of the Taoist idea. We, in every case, normally apply human-based qualities over normally happening examples. Be that as it may, recall it is likewise significant not to pursue better and better portrayals of these examples. To do so is to pursue down interminability.

Yin Yang is an arrangement of perceiving how to separate out examples in our life while additionally unwinding to acknowledge the general entire and complete nature of the Tao.

Yantra

Yantra is an enchanted chart utilized in the Indian religions and reasoning for love. It is utilized to help in contemplation and for the advantages of its mysterious implied forces dependent on Tantric writings and Hindu crystal gazing. It is a sort of mandala, which is an otherworldly image speaking to the universe.

In old-style Sanskrit, the word yantra signifies "instrument," "device," or "creation." It is gotten from the root word, yam, signifying "to help" or "to continue the quintessence of an item/idea."

Yantra alludes to any sort of instrument or machine that guides a venture. However, the importance has extended to allude to religious undertakings too.

Similarly, as mantras balance the body and psyche through sound, yantras give balance outwardly. They are geometric and incorporate botanical plans. The shapes are accepted to have an amazing calming impact on the psyche, as are utilized in yogic contemplation practice. Yantras are regularly connected with a specific god and might be worn as a charm.

Among the shapes utilized in yantras are squares, triangles, circles, and flower designs, however increasingly complex images might be utilized, each with significance. A lotus bloom symbolizes the chakra vitality focuses; a Bindu (speck) signifies both the purpose of creation and the limitless universe; a triangle means extroversion or manliness with an upward point, and inner-directedness or womanliness with a descending point; and a swastika symbolizes karma and thriving.

Yantra, Mantra, and Mandala

A Yantra is what could be compared to the Buddhist Mandala. It truly implies a 'machine' or a visual instrument that serves in contemplation. It is a microcosm of the universe. Yantra is different from Mantra in that, Yantra is the body or type of the god, while Mantra is the psyche.

How Are They Made?

Yantras are made through the amalgamation of different geometric structures and examples that show the mind the intensity of fixation and core interest. The drawing of a Yantra needs exactness, discipline, focus, tidiness, and accuracy. The visual structure of a Yantra actuates the correct side of the equator, which is visual and non-verbal.

Mantra

With profound practices like yoga and contemplation winding up progressively prevalent, it appears as though everybody is discussing mantras. Be that as it may, what precisely is a mantra and how are you expected to utilize it?

Sanskrit and Mantra

Getting to the old foundation, all things considered, mantra, at its center, is the premise of every single religious custom, sacred texts, and petitions. At the point when deliberately picked and utilized quietly, mantras are said to be able to help adjust your intuitive driving forces, propensities, and burdens. Mantras, when spoken or recited, direct the mending intensity of Prana (life power vitality) and, in conventional Vedic practices, can be utilized to empower and get to otherworldly conditions of cognizance. Mantra, as a profound practice, ought to be done all the time for a while for its ideal impacts to occur.

Toward the day's end, the mantra is intended to take you back to effortlessness. We live in such an unpredictable world that it is anything but difficult to lose all sense of direction in every one of the subtleties. Mantras can enable you to hover back to the oversimplified way to deal with life and spotlight on those things that motivate you and really satisfy you.

Reflection and Mantra

At the Chopra Center, where Primordial Sound Meditation is the favored reflection method, understudies are given a customized mantra, their Bija, which is the sound vibration the Universe was set aside a few minutes of their introduction to the world. This mantra is rehashed quietly again and again during the reflection practice to help the understudy in rising above the action of the psyche. The mantra is quiet and has no significance with the goal that the mind is not centered around a specific quality or result. It is just a vehicle that causes you to access uplifted degrees of mindfulness.

Mindfulness, in this unique circumstance, alludes to the capacity to focus on the decisions you make in your regular daily existence and perceive when something is not working so you can transform it. Numerous individuals face a great deal of pressure every day. You wake up, cook breakfast, feed the children, get them to class, get down to business, drink espresso for lunch, and consume the day. Before the part of the bargain, prepared to crash. At that point, you rehash the cycle the following day.

Building up a day by day contemplation practice causes you to develop an increasingly present, quiet, and adjusted lifestyle, which swells out into each other part of your life. Mantras can help take you back to that current situation with the psyche.

You've most likely heard the word mantra previously. Be that as it may, what you can be sure of is this is an otherworldly practice, and it is as old as it is significant.

We will investigate what mantras are, the different ways they can be utilized, and best of all — how you can give them something to do in your very own life for mind-blowing mending, strengthening, and change.

All in all, what is a mantra? Basically, it is a word, sound, syllable, or expression that has an incredible vibration reverberation.

They are utilized in reflection, yoga, and in the otherworldly practices of Buddhism, Hinduism, and Jainism.

You can utilize a mantra to think your vitality, open your chakras, and build up your mystic mindfulness. Otherworldly expresses, when opened, can raise your awareness. This training is so convincing and powerful. You have no clue where it could take you.

Individual mantra?

An individual mantra is an explanation that spurs and motivates you to be your best self.

With an individual mantra, you confirm the manner in which you need to carry on with your life. Also, it can help propel you to finish your objectives, both actually and expertly.

What Is Mantra Healing?

It has been demonstrated that reciting, music, and mantras strongly affect our cerebrum.

Mantras are fiery sound equations that moderate us down and permit us to see everything unmistakably. They give us a point of view.

Reciting quiets the body and actuates various normal substantial capacities and procedures. It can likewise help in mending the psyche and body from addictions, such as smoking or liquor. In addition, reciting can reinforce the resistant framework.

Reciting can lower pulse, lessen feelings of anxiety, increment hormone level execution, and abatement nervousness and gloom.

Who might have imagined that this straightforward practice could have such control?

Chapter 4: Yoga

Tips for Practicing Tantra Yoga

As you begin to embrace yoga as part of your tantric practices, there are a few things to always keep at the forefront of your mind. Don't lose sight of these key concepts, and you will experience maximum benefits from tantric yoga.

Breathing

In any tantric practice you pursue, your breath is your guide. On the mat or the mattress, it's very important to be attentive to your breathing and the breathing of your partner. Listening to your breath, and stabilizing it, makes all the difference in the practice. Often times, the stress and illness an individual feels are because the individual has lost track of how to breathe properly. It may seem strange at first because we all know the act of breathing as an unconscious process of the body; we don't need to remember to breathe. Except that we need to remember to breathe properly and deliberately. It's not uncommon for us to stifle our breathing and never really engage the diaphragm for a big breath into the stomach. Rather than take these bigger, more steady breaths, we take small breaths and keep our center from expanding. This delivers less oxygen to the blood, and the brain and improper breathing alone can affect our overall health, circulation, immune system, and energy levels. With practice, you will find your own steady and natural rhythm for breathing. Learn from yourself how this natural rhythmic breathing sounds and how it feels on the inhale and exhale. This way, when you're practicing the more ambitious tantric poses, you'll be able to recognize when your breath becomes uneven or unsteady, and it will be easier to restore yourself to the beneficial breath.

Listen and Communicate

You know now that one of the keys to tantra is to bring the spirit and the body into alignment and to allow for expansion and union with all around you. The way to do this is by quieting the mind and giving yourself the time to listen. An attentive listener is paying attention to what their own body is telling them. Is the breath steady and even? Is the body stretching too far in a posture? Too little? Which areas of the body need extra attention and expansion? What are the sensations the body registers in each pose? Go beyond your body, and listen to your thoughts; sit with them, work with them. If your mind is telling you the next posture will be too difficult, consider why that thought is coming to you. Is it founded on misconceptions and doubt, rather than experience? If it will be difficult, are you okay with that? Search your emotional state. Are you in a state of frustration in the pose, or are you at peace, despite the challenging movements? The more you practice listening to your own body, mind, and soul, the more you will be awakened to hear. Of course, if the practice is shared with your partner, listening goes beyond the self. Listening to your partner is just as critical in a tantric exercise. Not only should you be listening and aware of the signals and cues in your partner's body, mind, and heart, but you will need to practice gentle communication together. This strengthens the compassion and supports you each share together.

Be the Weaver

Take your practice to the next level. Going through the motions regularly and consistently will deliver numerous benefits, but you can, and should, use tantra to expand beyond the physical and explore your spiritual connection to yourself and your environment and the people within it. Through the practice of tantra, you begin to uncover your spiritual being. You begin to uncover the spiritual aspects of the physical world around you. As you do, the connections between yourself and your surroundings become recognizable. Aim for your best tantric life by allowing the expansion of your spiritual self to merge with your physical surroundings. This is, after all, exactly what is to be attained through tantric disciplines.

Let Go of Expectations

There are enough pressure and expectation from the outside world; you need not compound this with tantric work. Instead of practicing tantra for the sake of a particular outcome, practice tantra for the enjoyment of practicing. Let go of preconceived notions and expectations which may be within you, put there by you or the external world. Don't practice the yoga pose because you want it to be perfect; practice it because you enjoy the practice; you enjoy the meditative state, you enjoy your personal time with yourself. Don't enter into your sexual experience because you want to experience orgasm enter into it because you want to explore sensation. When you let go of expectations, you are free to enjoy the journey because no destination has been chosen. Support your partner in letting go of these expectations, as well. True liberation awaits you here.

Practice Regularly

It's true that practicing a few asanas here and there with no regularity will still benefit the body and the mind. However, the fullest benefits become yours with regular and consistent practice. As a comparison, think of going to the gym. You can go to the gym a handful of days out of the month, and you will still gain some benefit. But when you go to the gym daily, at a consistent time, for the entire month, the benefits will obviously be greater. You will build strength for running on the treadmill, and soon you may need to run faster, longer, or at a greater incline in order to challenge yourself. This is your expansion at the gym. Similarly, with regular and consistent tantric work, you will build strength for your discipline, and you will naturally cultivate your expansion this way. A challenging pose on day one will not be as challenging by day 30. A challenging sexual position you try for the first time, will not be so challenging when you've done it 30 times. Every aspect of your expansion comes from the regular and consistent practice of it.

Hatha Yoga

These tantric yoga poses are derived from the practice of Hatha yoga. Hatha yoga is one of the most popular methods of practicing yoga, especially in the western world. It's designed to quiet the mind and calm the soul. When you've practiced these poses outlined here, expand. Find other Hatha yoga movements, and you're curious to try and add them to your routine or replace a stale movement with a new one. Most any asana you find in

Hatha yoga will serve you in your pursuit of tantric living, and tantric sex.

Techniques for Enhancing Any Tantric Exercise

There are three techniques that will not only help you to develop a better overall sense of wellbeing, but they will also help you to remove worry, doubt, and anxiety from your day-to-day life. This, in itself, is an enormous benefit to your lifestyle, but the management or removal of these pressures will also be very evident in your love-making. These are some of the most widely studied and commonly applied techniques to help individuals to shift the way they think in order to develop positive patterns instead. These techniques are known as "the 3 Ms"- mindfulness, minimalism, and meditation. We'll take a look at the origins of each and how to apply these concepts in order to shift peacefully into your own expansion. Plus, you'll see examples of each of these as they apply to modify the negative and restrictive ideas your mind is conjuring, and what you can expect to see as a result of implementing these tools in your daily life. These concepts will help the individual to keep his or her mind from wandering, and it will help bring the wandering mind back to home-base when the thinker says to return. Use these approaches below to defeat overthinking, end negative automatic behaviors, and declutter your environment and your mind.

Mindfulness

Mindfulness, like simple living, is a concept that goes very far back through history but comes to the U.S. through relatively recent means. In the 1960s, the United States grew more familiar with Vietnamese Buddhist monk and activist, Thich Nhat Hanh. Hanh studied, practiced, and taught mindfulness, and in fact, taught at Princeton and Columbia University in the 60s. It is primarily through the teachings of Thich Nhat Hanh that mindfulness has found its way into Western culture. Thich Nhat Hanh taught in mindfulness to regularly take notice of where you are in your mental process. He also taught the importance of slowing down to live in the moment and practice the small daily pieces of life with extra-sensory focus. The teachings of Hanh were recognized by American medical professor and society founder of the University of Massachusetts Medical School, Jon Kabat-Zinn. For a time, Kabat-Zinn was a student of Hanh's and eventually went on to develop the study of mindfulness as we know it today.

Many of the techniques and practices used today in coaching and therapy, as well as personal practice, are rooted in the same two concepts: Bring yourself back. Refocus, recollect your thinking. When your mind begins to wander from the one thing you're doing, gently bring it back. Savor the moment you're in right now. Rather than wanting to rush through one thing to get to another, appreciate the step you're at in this very moment. If you're washing the dishes, your mind should stay on the one dish you're washing. You pay extra close attention to the experience of washing this one particular plate in this one particular moment. If your mind starts to slip and think about the next plate you'll wash, you gently bring it back to the plate you're holding and focus on, quite literally, the task at hand. Practicing mindfulness is a wonderful complement to practicing minimalism.

Both remind the individual that simple is better. If it feels too complicated, you can probably simplify it, whether it's a physical space or a mental attitude. Here are a few mindfulness techniques commonly used by practitioners and therapists, as well as self-practicing individuals. Keep in mind, they're all to do with the focus on the small and simple pieces of everyday life. They may seem mundane at first glance, but that's basically the point here. Something we might normally rush through is something we should fully observe and appreciate. That includes the moments that aren't so enjoyable. Sit in a chair, only. Find a chair and sit in it.

Don't do anything else. Sit in the chair only. Sit in that chair for about 5 minutes, and when your mind starts to wander, bring it back to the observation of the chair. How does it feel? How does it smell? What does it feel like? Hard or soft? Silky or leathery? What does your skin feel like on the chair? What does it sound like when you move in the chair? And when your mind begins to wander, gently bring it back to focus on the experience of sitting in a chair, and nothing else. Eat mindfully. When you're eating, alone or in a group, at home or the office, in any situation you find yourself eating practice mindfulness. Move your utensils more slowly than you normally might. Take a bite on your fork or spoon that will easily fit into your mouth without a struggle. Chew that piece of food more slowly than you normally might. Pay closer attention to the textures and flavors.

Put your utensil down while you chew. Take a sip of water after swallowing your food. Engage the senses. This can be something as simple as enjoying the smell of the soap or shampoo you use in the shower, or something as extreme as skydiving. There's a wide range of activities from one to the other, and you're sure to find comfort somewhere between them. Give your senses a new thrill. Visit a new city or town. Listen to new music. Rent a car just to switch it up. Try a food you've never had. Find ways of igniting the senses. Listen, and nothing else. When someone is talking, give your full attention to them.

Meditation

Meditation is an ancient practice that dates back as early as 5000BC, and perhaps even further. Thus, it's difficult to say with any accuracy when and where meditation began. What's easily known is that meditation began to make its way into the United States at the end of the 1800s, as the western world became familiar with India through Great Britain.

At a time in society when the paranormal and the occult were all the rage, meditation, and really any exotic alternative that broke norms and challenged taboos, fit right in. Meditation on a large scale can represent a religious devotion. Meditation on a smaller scale can offer a decrease in perceptual stress and anxiety, and improved health, especially of the heart and circulatory system. It's recommended that you meditate for as little as 10 minutes each day. Meditating for a longer period of time can be beneficial too, but for many, it creates too much resistance, and only 10-20 minutes is achievable. A routine practice of 10 minutes or more, at least once a day, can have a significant impact on you physically and mentally.

There are many people who think meditation doesn't work for them, or they cannot do it. This is an unfortunate misconception. In almost every case of this, the individual has been misinformed about what meditation is, and what's to be expected. When the individual is freed from the restrictive thoughts of what meditation must be, they are able to enjoy its benefits without resistance. There are many different types of meditation, but in one form or another, most forms of meditation focus on creating a silence in mind.

In whichever form of meditation you practice, this usually means that you become quiet and still and focus on an external stimulus like the sound of your breathing or the sound of the wind or water. When your mind begins to wander, you bring it back to the moment and refocus on the sound of your breath, or the wind, or the water. Let's take a look at several types of meditation that can be easily practiced almost anywhere by almost anyone. Pay attention to which forms of meditation sound comfortable to you and test one out today.

Kindness Meditation

In this meditation exercise, you sit in a peaceful and quiet location for about 10 minutes with your eyes closed. During this time, you keep your mind on only one thought. The thought is usually a message of loving-kindness you want to send to someone. For example, let's say a friend has a broken leg and you're hoping for them to recover soon. To perform a kindness meditation, prepare a short basic sentence that expresses your love for your friend and your desire to see them well again. As you meditate, repeat this phrase as a sort of mantra, all the while trying to elicit the positive emotional feelings of seeing your friend well again. When the mind wanders, bring it back to this mantra.

Progressive Relaxation

In this meditation exercise, you sit in a calm and quiet environment and become still and soft. Typically, you would begin by slowing the breath and listening to it, concentrating on the sound of it. After about a minute or so, you focus on one small aspect of your being with the goal of relaxing it. For example, let's say it's time to relax your jaw. Wiggle your jaw and stretch it out for a moment. Imagine the tiny muscles and nerves in your chin relaxing. Imagine your tongue relaxing. Move your tongue around in your mouth, and feel it relax. As you relax each part, you move to another, slowly relaxing pieces of yourself from head to toe. If you intend to practice meditation for longer than 10 minutes, this is an excellent one to start with. It keeps the analytical mind focused on the task, and the extra relaxation makes it easy to stay in this meditation for upwards of 20 minutes.

Kundalini Yoga

This yoga practice doubles as a meditation practice, and the individual experiences peace of mind through focus, and physical health benefits as well. To practice Kundalini, you would learn a set of poses or movements that you would blend together. Each time you restart the movements, you focus on making them as perfect as you can. When the mind wanders, you bring it back to your form. The set of movements usually includes 4 - 8 poses that start over at the completion of each set. There are, of course, many other forms of meditation, and if none of these sound as if they'll suit you, don't give up on meditation. Consider what it is you're looking for in an effective meditative exercise and then use other resources to find the form of meditation that will best suit you. By adding as little as 10 minutes of meditation to your day, you're reducing stress and anxiety. You're quieting the mind and training it to know that obsessive negative thought patterns are not the only thought patterns you have at your disposal. Allowing yourself to rest the body and mind simultaneously for just 10 minutes a day promotes emotional health and enhances self-worth and self-actualization. Meditation is an excellent tool for lengthening the attention span and improving memory, and it can actually reduce memory loss for seniors as they age. You can look forward to more control over your thoughts and emotions with 10 minutes to realign and focus.

Chapter 5: Tantric Techniques

Tips for sexier sex huh, is this at all possible? Oh Yes, It is Possible! Enhancing the orgasms that you do have and increasing possibilities for more through Tantric Positioning might sound complicated but anyone can do it. It is just exploring the best positions for you and your partner to help improve your sex life.

To begin, It is Courage, Bravery, Sexual Confidence along with the ability and willingness to act on it. If you have any hang ups or inhibitions about being naked with the light on or certain sexual positions the time to let that go is right now.

Letting go of any hangups you might have is the best way to get sexual satisfaction and the benefits that come along with it. Limits and restrictions are not good bedfellows for great sex and are often an indication there is some inner psychological hurdle.

Anything that prevents us from giving and receiving sexual pleasure between two consenting adults is keeping you from maximizing your potential for new and innovative orgasms. It is often said the road to true sexual freedom and a healthy happy sexual self-esteem is to 'responsibly' let yourself go and explore the boundaries(an important note: This is almost always achieved through faithful monogamy).

There is absolutely nothing wrong or 'dirty' about any sexual position between two Consenting loving adults. It is a natural expression of love and feeling the release of your instincts and desires. We all want to be more confident sexually and the way to make that happen is through not allowing anything to stand in the way of our sexual ambition.

Enough about that now right? We are all liberated and ready for fearlessly exploring our real sexual well-being, intimacy on the highest levels possible. We are ready to explore the absolute best Tips for Sexier Sex by enhancing Our Orgasms to be the best they can be and always improving.

Of course you realize this means overcoming any fears of, or worries about, trying some new things. Embarking on the journey of new sensations and opening yourself up to new ideas about sex. It involves a lot of trust. It is beyond worth it in the end and is why so many couples are successful in their relationships.

Finding a true connection and love begins and end with great sex. A healthy happy satisfying sex life is the one crucial vital element in a passionate and loving relationship. There is more to a couple than sex but that is the one thing they have that solidifies their "togetherness." It is what makes them 'In' Love and that's how you get to have great orgasms.

Orgasm Enhancing Positions

Coital Alignment Technique - (C.A.T.)

For me this brings the missionary position back to life. It is always good no matter what but when you approach a position with the feminine aspect in mind its improved by a thousand fold. If she is more apt to be pleased by this old-time favorite position then so much the better and that is what C.A.T. is all about.

Coital Alignment Technique requires the base of the penis and pelvic bone to stimulate the clitoris while thrusting with a patient rhythm. Constant clitoral stimulation is the calling card of C.A.T. Subtle but crafty full body movements with You Guessed it Constant Clitoral Stimulation is the best way to describe and achieve C.A.T..

The number of positions available are endless and this is in no way any attempt to list them. The few named here are just the beginning and more geared towards orgasm friendly with relative ease. Though they still require practice.

Please Stand Up, Put your hands and Face up against the Wall. Any position that allows easy access for manual clitoral stimulation while copulating is going to be a prime candidate for being an Orgasm Enhancing Position. This one is perfect and underutilized by many couples.

The woman standing puts her palms against a wall and then leans forward while tensing (or arching the waist) and sticks out her bottom. This allows the man to come in from behind and can easily kiss while with his hand massages a swirling motion rub to her clitoris. Such graphic details!

Tantric Lovemaking - Tantra is very hard to describe in short order. Entire volumes have been written covering only certain aspects of the vast topic of Tantra Sex. Tantra is a subject beyond that of sex but a religious, spiritual practice and Hindu Philosophy.

Is learning how to harness your particular sexual energy and transfer share and deliver it over to another as a power. This is a spiritual power of sexual depth and complete control through letting go. Liberation often ending in true sexual satisfaction and deep connection between the two love-makers.

Ending the tips to sexier sex and enhancing orgasms through Tantric Positioning with a small list from the eternal amount of Tantric style lovemaking is efficient enough for me.

Soul-gazing- staring into each others' eyes.

Passionate Caresses- Obviously erotic message is always a great preemptive technique to begin with.

Yab-Yum- Classic tantra position of sitting Indian Style with woman on top her legs around him. You are facing each other.

Laying of Hands- During sex whenever you are close to climax, lay your hands over your lovers' heart to signal it to them and stare at each other during the climax.

Pranayama or Regularisation of Breath- Breathing in unison together and also creating a kind of yin-yang rhythm together. It will come natural and all of a sudden become a bigger part of your sex by offering more control—Ultimately bringing on shared or simultaneous orgasms.

Orgastic Circulation of Light- Creative visualization is an advance technique that can drastically increase the intensity of your togetherness. Both of you will creatively visualize the same thing. Usually a sphere, a ball of glowing light between you while making love. It can rise and descend between you changing color at different intervals.

Tips to Start Tantric Touching

Many people take lessons in Tantric lovemaking and these classes are all about the positions. But this section is about Tantric love but not the sex positions like most of the Tantric love lessons on Internet talk about. Tantric love making is about connecting with your partner in heart, body, mind and spirit. And for enabling everyone to achieve this, TANTRIC TOUCHING has to be revealed. What is tantric touching? Why emphasize on it?

Tantric touching is to touch or physically connect with your partner in a deeper and more spiritual way. With the hectic lives we all lead today, it is so amazing how many couples do not even take the time to connect with each other via a simple loving touch. Well I can leave you to be one of those people. But reading this part will teach you a few Tantric touching tips that will deepen your sexual intimacy with your love lady.

Tantric Touching 101 Tips

You have to MAKE time for Tantric touching. You can not keep leading your hectic life and complain you don't have time for your lady. MAKING time is most essential. If you can schedule a meeting at work and she can schedule an appointment at the beauty parlor, then you two can certainly make time for one another. Let me help you, get you calendars out right away and block an hour this Friday or the weekend to just be with one another. These dates are best as there is always something about a weekend that makes your minds and bodies relax.

Prepare yourselves properly. Now if you thing just sitting casually in front of each other and starting to touch is not what I am on about here. Its not like the the effects of Tantric touching are just going to magically come without your special efforts. You both have to prime yourselves a bit. You want primer tips? Here

Sit down and have a nice cup of herbal tea together.

Take a walk hand in hand.

*Take a shower together, a bath is even better.

The main reason for these primers was that you have to get your body accustomed to relax in each others presence.

Prepare a Tantric touch area. If you think you can actually start a session of Tantric touching just any where in your home, then stop thinking that way right away. This is a practice that has to reach out to you spiritually, so you need a quiet, and peaceful area. I recommend both of you take some time in preparing the area for the touching session. You should do it together to heighten your experience. If you do not want to take it together, and are a bit on the non romantic sides, then I reckon you do it alone when your wife/girlfriend is in the bath. Now you do not know what to do to prepare a touch area? Here you go---Place a nice soft rug on the floor and put a lot of pillows over it, this is so that your bodies are nicely cushioned. Then play some SOFT music and light some scented candles or burn some scented oils. Candles are loved by most women and scents we all know what they mean to women. But make sure you don't make the smell too strong. It has to be a WHIFF of something nice and not a SCENT ASSAULT. If you have rose petals ready for your encounter, then scatter them too on the rug.

Free her inhibitions. When she is ready to join you, you can ask her to lie down on her back and close her eyes. The best is if she is wearing a lingerie or nightgown. Let her not feel uncomfortable or vulnerable. If she is not then in stead of asking her to close her eyes, just simply blind fold her.

Drink in her whole presence. Before touching her, step back and just observe her beauty. Just admire your woman. Start with the tips of her toes and work your eyes up her whole body till you reach the very of her head. Do not make the mistake of looking up and down with the goal of critiquing or even trying to find her 'best parts'. Simply preview her as a really exquisite painting by a master.

Speak your desire. Mind you, you still have not started touching her. Now you have to start by telling her sweetly how you just LOVE certain parts of her body more than ever before. This is bound to come out of your mouth as you will be looking at her like the best piece of art by the master, the God himself. Do not hold back and let out all your positive comments, even if they sound LUSTFUL. This will make her feel loved, and cherished and yes, a bit HORNY too. This comes from personal experience so you do not have to hesitate in this.

Start touching her. Start physical contact with her body and it does not matter where you touch first but the best is to start with SMALL TOUCHES. I'll give you an example here, start with touching her toes with only just your finger tips, in stead of holding with your whole hands and grabbing her butt right away. No matter how small your touch will be, make it firm, as your goal here is not to tickle her after all. Give this part a bit of time before you move on to firmer, bigger touches and to the rest of the body.

Pay attention to her reactions. Take notice as to how she is reacting to your sexual touches. Is she relaxed? Too relaxed? or is she seemingly tensed? If she is too relaxed then your touches have to be FIRMER. Let me give you a personal experience tip here, try firmer definitely but make your touches a bit more naughty. If you find her a bit too tensed then you might be actually pushing her to an early sexual release. Ease her up a bit so she is not pushed over the edge. Now there can also be a situation that you are unable to find out how she is feeling about the way you are touching her. This is usually the case when the two of you have not spent enough time together for quite sometime now. Here are some ways to help you KNOW how she feels about your sexual touches:

Is she making noises? What type of noises? Sure you might have heard similar noises before for different reasons while making love when you were having a better sex life than now. So when you know what does a particular noise mean, you will know if she is enjoying it or no.

Her facial feature! For example, are her brows relaxed or tensed. Now for different women the brow tensed or relaxed means different. Now personally I know that when my lady frowns a bit she is LOVING what I am doing to her. Now you have to certainly have the prior experience with your woman to engage in Tantric touching, so that you know her expressions just too well.

How is her skin? Are they bit flushed? are they cool with goose bumps on them? Tip here is to light bit more candles and lather some warm oil to increase the temperature if she is cool.

The key to Tantric touching is that you have to pay COMPLETE attention to how she is reacting, so then you can react accordingly. You have to just keep one thing in mind, you have to make her feel relaxed in her mind, body and spirit. Use this as the primer for making love so it would do well if the Tantric touching session is a success. Remember this is love and not for those who care only about lust. These and several other techniques are for LOVE MAKING and not lustful sexual encounter. This helps you in creating a spiritual bond with your partner, which, mark my words will forever keep improving your relationship with your partner.

Tantric Techniques For Ecstatic Lovemaking

When was the last time you can remember feeling totally ecstatic during lovemaking? Has it been weeks, months or years? Maybe you've never had the opportunity to know what sexual ecstasy really feels like, until you've tried these 3 tantric techniques...

1. Tantric Eye-Gazing This tantric technique can instantly create intimate connections with your lover. In a standing or seated position, place your left hand over your partner's right hand and your right hand over their left. Synchronize your breath with your lover's and as you do, slowly allow your hands to rise on the inhale and descend on the

exhale. Continue breathing at the same rhythm, looking softly into your lover's left-eye, as she looks at yours.

In the Celtic tradition, it is believed that the eyes are the "gateway to the soul", unifying two souls as one, while connecting people together through many lifetimes. In tantra, eye-gazing is often used before or during lovemaking to enhance the emotional, spiritual and physical bond with your lover. Practiced frequently, it can lead to powerful states of ecstasy.

2. Tantric Breathing The effects of stress and living in a fast-paced society can have a tremendous impact on the way we breathe. Most people don't pay attention to their breath and tend to be very shallow breathers. When you are learning how to have tantric sex, the first thing you start with is deep abdominal breathing, which is the most natural way to cultivate prana or life force energy. Tantric breathing is also essential to sexual health. Not only does it prolong intercourse, but it can enhance and multiply sexual pleasure for both partners.

There are many ways to practice tantric breathing. You can do it alone or during lovemaking. Simply start by placing your hand on your navel and inhale, counting slowly to 4. Notice as your abdomen begins to rise. Then, exhale to the count of 4, while sighing out noisily. Continue to breathe in this manner during sex.

3. Cultivating Sexual Energy Many tantric techniques teach sexual control in order to cultivate sexual energy. Sexual energy is the most powerful human force and most people tend to waste it readily through frequent ejaculation and orgasm. When we cultivate sexual energy, we deliberately bring ourselves to the peak of orgasm and then stop before we climax, drawing the energy up with our breath, to the crown of our heads and back down again. This natural energy, remains inside us, connecting our mind, body and spirit. It can help us achieve heightened states of ecstasy, creativity and serve as a healing force.

During lovemaking, when you and your partner are about to reach climax, stop by contracting your genitals, as though you are stopping the flow of urine. Then, close your eyes and breathe into your belly, about 2 inches below the navel. As you exhale, focus on the crown of your head. Repeat this breath 4 times. On the fourth breath, gently open your eyes and allow the sexual energy to flood into your heart and spread through you from the top of your head, all the way down to the tips of your toes. Let it fill you to overflowing.

Chapter 6: Tantra Sex Positions

Right now, you will find out about various Tantric sex positions and procedures that you can use for spicing up your sexual coexistence.

The Sidewinder

This position is enlivened from the yoga position of a similar name, and this procedure takes into account deep entrance. It likewise accommodates the couple to keep in touch. For playing out this method, the lady should rest on her side and supports the heaviness of her chest area with the assistance of her hands. She should lift one of her legs and place it on her darling's shoulder while the other leg is lying on the bed. A variety of this equivalent position is that then again, the man can rest behind the lady and enter his partner from behind.

The Yab Yum

The Yab Yum position is viewed as probably the best situation for having tantric sex. It is a genuinely simple situation to perform, and it takes into consideration synchronous climaxes. This position helps in animating quite a few places. Likewise, the man's hands happen to be free right now, and he can touch his darling's body. However, he sees fit since the couple would confront one another. It takes into consideration enthusiastic kisses also. The man should sit leg over leg on the bed or some other agreeable surface and hold his back straight. The lady should straddle him and fold her legs over his lower back. It takes into account delayed here and there developments that can help the couple in accomplishing an all-around planned climax.

The Latch

This posture permits the man to get a decent see his sweetheart's face and the other way around. This is an extremely attractive posture and aides in pleasuring both the partners. For playing out this procedure, the lady should be situated on a high stage like a table or even the kitchen counter. She will then need to recline and adjust her upper-middle and her head with the assistance of her hands by inclining onto her elbows. The man should remain between her separated legs and enter her. This is one represent that doesn't need to be limited to the room and is ideal for an off the cuff cavort.

The Butterfly

This method is accepted to allow both the partners to achieve a significant level of rapture and takes into consideration deep entrance. For playing out this system, the young lady should rest on the table so that her butt lies at the edge of the table, and the man should help lift her lower back marginally off the table and afterward place both her legs over his shoulders. Her vagina would be free for him to infiltrate while remaining in the middle of her legs. Since her legs are shut together, this fixes the vaginal waterway and gives a tight fit. The man should enter her while her butt is in midair.

The Double Decker

This is an amazingly suggestive posture and will help in accomplishing a climax, no problem at all. The man will likewise be given a decent perspective on all the activity that is going on down there, and his hands will likewise have unlimited access to lay with his sweetheart's butt. This position is very enabling for ladies since they have all the control here. For playing out this system, the man should sit on the bed while his legs are collapsed under his body. The lady will then need to confront away from him and place her feet on either side of her darling while her feet are set level superficially to give her some help. When she has brought down herself onto his erect penis, then she will just need to begin moving advances and in reverse or can even decide on a here and there movement. The man should basically kick back and have fun.

The Last Place Anyone Would Want To Be

This is an extraordinary posture since it permits both the gatherings to have a similar measure of control and ooze a similar measure of pressure for having a great sexual encounter. People will have an equal balance right now. For playing out this represents, the man should sit on the bed and support his chest area with his knees. He will then need to move the lower some portion of his legs in reverse and place them marginally separated. The lady will then need to expect a similar position, yet she will do as such while confronting ceaselessly from him, and her run would be squeezing into his scrotum and her back against his chest. Her legs would be joined and afterward set in the space that is accessible between his legs, and the man should enter her from behind. For this situation to be compelling, both the partners should remain as near to one another as could reasonably be expected.

Skiff

This position is a slight adjustment of the lady on top position. Right now, bodies should be situated so that both the partners will find a good pace great take a gander at one another's face while occupied with the demonstration. For playing out this, the man should sit down on a seat that can marginally twist in reverse. The lady will then need to put herself on his lap and afterward place her legs on either side of the seat. The young lady should fire an allover development without anyone else, or her partner can help her by setting his hand under her bum and helping her move in an upwards and downwards way.

The Mermaid

This is a somewhat fluctuated adaptation of the butterfly, and it takes into consideration a more solace and better hold. Right now, man can play with his darling's feet. Remember that feet are viewed as one of the most touchy and erogenous pieces of a lady's body. For playing out this method, the lady should expect a similar situation as she did in the butterfly. However, her butt ought to be propped with the assistance of a pad. Her legs should loosen up and ought to be at a 90-degree edge. The man should stand near the table and infiltrate her.

Tsunami

This posture is very agreeable, and it is a sensual treat. This will knock your socks off. This posture is a slight alteration of the exemplary minister style. Right now, the lady should expect the job that a man, as a rule, does in the teaching style. For playing out this, the man should rest level on his back, and his arms should be put close by. The lady should lie over him, and the man should embed his penis into her vagina. The lady should totally loosen up her legs with the goal that they are resting on his. Her palms ought to be put on his lower arm for giving her some help. The lady will then need to begin moving her pelvis in an upward and descending development.

Lap Dance

This is a great posture for a man to encounter his darling's body in the entirety of its magnificence. His hands will be allowed to meander around her body, and he can do what he needs. The lady will face away from him as she would have, had she been giving him a lap move. For playing out this represents, the man should sit down on a seat, and his back should be kept straight. The lady will then sit on his lap and parity herself by setting her hands on his upper thighs or even his stomach. She will then need to lift herself gradually and place the backs of her calves and brings down herself onto his penis. Another variety of this would be that the lady should bring down herself onto his penis while confronting her darling, and this will give him a serious decent perspective on her bosoms. He can choose to prod and play with them for whatever length of time that he satisfies.

Pretzel

This is another representation that is satisfying to take a gander at and even simple to expect. This will cause the couple to feel incredibly attractive. For playing out this procedure, the couple should stoop before one another. The man should move advances, and the lady will fold her arms over him. The lady will then lift herself up and place her left leg by her darling's correct foot; her foot will confront downwards. The man will then need to put his left leg close to her correct foot. When taken a gander at a couple occupied with this posture, they look like a pretzel, an extremely provocative and mouth-watering pretzel.

The Spread

This is an essential and amazingly hot position. This permits the lady to get incredible delight since it lets her stroke her sweetheart and permits him the entrance to joy her. For playing out this system, the lady should sit at the very edge of the couch or even the bed and spread her legs separated. The man will then need to remain in the middle of her legs and infiltrate her. She can draw nearer to him and kiss him while his hands have the entrance to her full body.

The Entwine

This posture looks intense and difficult to copy. However, then it very well may be pleasurable if it's done appropriately. This posture is tastefully engaging. For playing out this strategy, the couple should sit near one another and face each other. The man should put his legs on either side of his partner. The lady will then need to lift both of her legs and place them on either side of her sweetheart's sides under his arms. The man's upper arms will secure the lady's legs, and the lady will then need to lift her upper arms and place them over his elbows. The man will then lift his legs and place them over her hands. This does sound very muddled, isn't that right? All the exertion that goes into it will merit your time and energy.

The G-force

This is maybe one of the most blazing tantric sex presents there is. This is the piece de opposition of all sex presents. The man has full oversight over his darling right now, both the people included will get extraordinary delight from this posture. For playing out this position, the lady should rest on her back on the bed, and the man must bow by her legs. He will then gradually lift her middle off the bed, so she's offsetting herself with her head and her shoulders put on the bed. The man can extend her legs at a 90-degree edge or infiltrate her, or he can likewise pull them separated and place her feet just beneath his chest and enter her.

The Waterfall

Right now, the lady should put her hand on her sweetheart's penis and afterward let her fingertips brush his scrotum gradually and tenderly. It is a smart thought to use some ointment for making it progressively pleasurable. Her hands should be set on either side of his gonads, and afterward, she should gradually slide her hands up till they arrive at the touchy tip of his penis. When this is done, the lady should give the man some time to chill off, and he will then need to respond to the administration he got. The man needs to cup his sweetheart's vagina and touch all her delicate spots. He should slide his hands over her clitoris and her external vaginal lips.

The Snake

For this, the lady should gradually extend the pole of her sweetheart's penis with one of her hands and let the other hand follow little circles directly under the leader of the pole. This is like giving slow and delicate handwork. Proceed with these movements a clockwise way, and afterward, once you arrive at the leader of the penis move to anticlockwise heading. Keep this up for whatever length of time that your sweetheart can suffer it.

Tantric Triangle of Touch

The lady should rests on her back and spread her legs somewhat and twist them at the knee. The man will then need to embed his list and center finger into her vagina and marginally twist them upwards till they make a come here development. This will give the ideal incitement to her G-Spot. This will make her groan in delight. While doing this, he should put the palm of his other hand on her lower midriff and apply a little delight. This consolidated incitement will rapidly push her off the edge.

The Teeter-Totter

There is nothing remotely guiltless about this specific teeter-totter. This is exceptionally suggestive. The lady should rest on her back on the bed, and her pelvis should be somewhat tilted upwards. A pad can be propped under her pelvis for doing as such. The man will then need to lift her feet and tenderly overlap them with the goal that her knees are laying on her bosoms, and the bottoms of her feet are touching his chest. This position permits unhindered access to a lady's vagina and the upward tilt will guarantee that he hits her G-Spot each time he pushes into her.

Tub Tangle

Get your man to lean back in a tub that is loaded up with water, and the lady should straddle him while her back is confronting him. When his penis has entered her, he should sit up, so you both are confronting one another. Then she should fold her legs over him, and he will do likewise with the goal that their elbows are under their partner's knees. Clutch each other as firmly as you can and start an influencing to and fro movement. This allows for some enthusiastic kissing.

Love Triangle

The lady should rest on her back on the floor or the bed, and afterward, she should lift her left advantage into the air. Her correct legs ought to be loosened up to her correct side, with the end goal that both her legs are lying opposite to one another. She will then need to move her correct hand and catch her correct knee and form a triangle on the bed with the use of her correct leg and her correct hand. The man should hunch a little and enter her while holding her knee. This position would give the man better pelvic control and furthermore the chance of touching from multiple points of view as you would need to. A slight variety can be added to this posture by requesting that the man pivot his hips in a roundabout movement while pushing into the lady; this will push the couple to their verge.

Presently and Zen

This posture can be used for giving a snapshot of relief from the approaching climax. Tantric sex isn't tied in with discovering speedy discharge; it is tied in with enjoying the experience. What's a better approach to do as such, than to control yourself directly before arriving at the final turning point. When you feel that you or your partner may be near climaxing, enjoy a couple of moments and reprieve liberated from the position that you both are in. The man can just roll onto his side and remain inside his partner at the same time. This position just requests a snapshot of a break. Slow pushing is passable. However, if you feel that you are going to climax, then pause for a minute, delay, maybe appreciate a tad of kissing and touching before proceeding with where you had given up. This position gives the genuinely necessary closeness during the sex to make the entire experience additionally adoring and healthy.

Torrid Tug-of-War

The lady should sit leg over leg on the floor or some other agreeable surface and afterward gradually sink onto his erect penis and fold her legs over his back. This position will permit the couple to confront one another, and this implies you can grasp each other's elbows for offering some help and incline toward the bearing endlessly from your partner. This resembles playing a round of shy back-and-forth. If you both happen to be adaptable, then one partner can tilt their heads back and lean in reverse, away from the other partner. This position will take into account the arrangement of your bodies, and it will cause you to associate with your partner. It frames a close association and aides in gathering speed. Both the partners find a good pace player right now. The entrance can be controlled, on the other hand, by the partners.

The Python

The man should rest right now, and his legs ought to be kept near one another while his arms are resting by his sides. The lady should bring down herself onto his penis and mount him gradually. When the man has entered her, then she can extend herself above with the goal that she's laying completely on his body. Both of your bodies would be superbly adjusted, and you can get a handle on one another's hands for gathering some speed and furthermore for offering some help. The lady will then need to gradually lift her middle off his with the goal that it nearly appears to be a snake that is ready to strike. She can push against his feet for including some greater development. You will both be touching each other completely, and her bosoms would rub against his chest, your hands would be gotten a handle on firmly, and his thighs would rub against hers. It takes into consideration a deep entrance. However, it additionally takes into account clitoral incitement. Since the couple would confront one another, this takes into account some enthusiastic kissing too. All the erogenous zones in the body would be animated.

Chapter 7: Tantric Masturbation

Man's secret pleasure point

Male masturbation is described as the act of a man pleasuring himself by either touching or stimulating his penis, nipples, testicles, and other erogenous zones in his body. These self-pleasuring techniques usually carry on to the point of ejaculation or orgasm, and it is done purely to satisfy his sexual pleasure. This can be done either solo or when you're in private or as part of the foreplay leading up to sex with their partner, although most of the time, masturbation typically happens when the man is alone. As a man, masturbation can help you deal with anxieties, understand your sexual preferences, your body, improve your endurance during sex, and generally keeps you happy.

Woman's secret pleasure point

Masturbation can be just as life-changing for a woman's sex life as it can be for a man. Many women struggle with body issues and poor self-image, but masturbation is a way of overcoming that and learning to love your body as it is. When you know how to pleasure yourself, it makes it easier to guide your partner about what they need to go to take your orgasms to the next level. Self-love is important for a woman because it can deeply affect your intimacy with your partner when you're not comfortable in your own skin. If you haven't spent a lot of time pleasuring yourself before this, it's never too late to start.

First, get to know your body better by holding a mirror between your legs to see what your partner sees when they are touching you or giving you oral sex. Take a good look at what you look like down there. This is you. This is your body. Now, start to feel around a little bit, massaging your vulva and locating your clitoris. Play around the area and observe the way your body responds to the touch. Some areas will feel oh so good while others will feel very, VERY good. You want to keep the sensation going on the "very good" areas.

Hand tricks to give extreme pleasure

Masturbation is often thought of as a solo act, but it could be surprisingly pleasurable to do this with your partner. Masturbation is an intimate thing, and sharing this moment with someone you care about can bring you closer together as a couple. Mutual masturbation can be an incredible moment shared between you and your partner. For the man, watching his partner masturbate is probably high on his sexual wish list. It may not be as high on the list for the woman, but you may be surprised at how arousing it could be. As a bonus, you may each learn something new about your partner's arousal process. Some women may never even have seen a man ejaculate in real life other than is watched in porn films. Men, ejaculating in front of your partner is a very intimate act, and surprisingly enough, many women find it arousing not only physically but mentally and emotionally.

Face-to-Face

This position can be pulled off in a few ways, depending on how you and your partner like to do it. Begin by lying down on your side, facing your partner, and gazing into their eyes. The closer you are; the greater the intimacy and intensity of the moment. Touch yourself the way you would if you were masturbating alone and watch your partner's face start to change as they pleasure themselves too. It's a great time to throw in some dirty talk here. Keep this going until you both climaxes, perhaps even try attempting to orgasm at the same time.

Don't Ask

Instead of asking for sex, show your partner that you're in the mood instead. This tip works best for women, and without saying a word, position yourself provocatively comfortably and make sure he's got a good view. Place two fingers in an inverted V straddling your clitoris. This hand position is good for encouraging your orgasm. Throw yourself into your masturbation session with abandon and watch his face start to change as continues watching you pleasure yourself.

Stimulating His Testicles

This secret is key to giving your man some of the best orgasms of his life. This secret is in the testicles and knowing how to use them as a secret weapon of pleasure. Cup your partner's testicles gently and begin stroking them softly. Hold them and very lightly pull them towards you (be gentle here because his testicles will be sensitive to your touch). To double the pleasure, give him fellatio while you do this, it's going to drive him crazy as the stimulation of both his penis and his balls at the same time will make it hard for him not to finish right then and there. The warmth and moisture of your mouth around his penis, along with his testicles being gently rubbed, will lead straight to orgasmic bliss.

Chapter 8: Tantric Massage

Tantra massage is one of the most unique forms of massaging. It's also something that's not readily available everywhere you go cause of the fact that it demands a certain form of specialization and professionalism. The masters who perform these massages own both the basic and advanced principles and skills needed to perform tantra and meditation. The massage starts off with ancient Asian and Tantric rituals, followed by a state of meditation, focusing body and mind to allow complete physical and spiritual access.

It's important to keep in mind that a tantra massage is not there to drive away pain and fatigue but to allow your hidden mystic energy to ooze out through your pores, bringing your body and soul in absolute synchronization with the universe. When adding or incorporating music to your tantric massage, make sure to pick something in the line of tantra or meditation. Records like these are rare but available.

Tantra Massage uses light, bodily and leisurely strokes to channel the energy and boost your body's sensitivity to a different world. Medium to hard pressure may also be wished to apply to sides of your spine, but other than that stick to soft and sensual using only movements in which energy arrives and departs your body.

Oils, lotion, and creams all work well with tantric massages but try staying clear of scented oils or lotions which may distract and draw your attention to other things. The two basic necessity for this message is music and a state of meditation. Tantric massage has proven to work for injuries, illnesses and even couples can take advantage of the amazing healing powers to increase closeness and spiritual well being. Tantra uses fundamentals like love, compassion, and trust instead of sex.

There are various ways to learn and practice Tantra. Among all the ways, tantric massage is the most resulting one. A good tantra massage includes several other components than only the message. Proper meditation, tantric yoga, breathing, relaxation, and effective sexual techniques are the other components of such a message.

A tantra massage, unlike other massage techniques, requires an emotional bonding between the giver and the receiver. It is quite natural that a stranger cannot satisfy a person in any way like a familiar person can do. Therefore, it is a good idea to avoid all the commercials that claim to give an effective tantric massage. Proper trust and proper intimacy are the two basic things of various tantra rituals, exercises, and tantra techniques.

A person re?uires should do certain things for a good tantra massage. First of all, the message should take place in such an environment that is useful to offer complete relaxation of both body and mind. The place should also be free from any kind of disturbances. The place better is detached from any kind of contact with the outside world.

The surface on which the message would take place is e?ually important like the environment. Since comfort and relaxation are the most sought after things, a soft mattress, mat, or even a fresh sheet can do the work. Towels offering proper support to the knees and neck area are a must. Avail great ?uality massage oil made of herbs, which can enhance the effectiveness of the message. There are certain other things which can boost the level of relaxation attained through tantric massage. Mild incense, soft pious music, and candlelight can definitely do the magic.

The receiver should recline on his her stomach as the massage starts. A gentle foot massage is an ideal thing to start the message. Gradually, the treatment should shift towards the neck and shoulder area. The important pressure points that are present in the neck and shoulder area can offer the best relaxation throughout the body if treated with proper massage strokes. The back area is the next place where the masseur should focus on. The joints and the muscular areas should receive proper care to help the receiver get rid of all the stress. When the back area is complete, the receiver should slowly turn around. This will help the masseur take care of the front area.

A person should keep in mind that tantric massage is not only popular for providing the receiver's body with a great level of relaxation. Tantra is equally popular for the energy that it can restore in the body of a person. So, as a person feel relaxed after the massage, he/she can also gather an adequate amount of energy for the upcoming time. This energy helps balance the chakras - several energy centers shared through the central axis of a body. These chakras, once properly energized, can help the recipient unleash various emotional as well as physical benefits.

A tantric massage goes perfect when followed by sexual activity. But, such activities should follow half an hour after the message. Therefore, keep these guidelines in mind and this weekend, you can offer your partner something that every human being looks for - ultimate relaxation.

Transformation Through Tantra Meditation

Tantra meditation takes cognizance of the fact that there is no such thing as mindless sex. Your tantra teacher will instruct you in honing the mind into a highly evolved, powerful sexual tool.

With tantra meditation, intimate partners learn to approach the sexual act with complete mindfulness. With tantric meditation, sex is no longer just carnal lust and gratification but becomes something spiritual. Inhibitions, reservations, and self-doubt dissolve under the advance of complete awareness of the act, the desire that drives it and the object of desire. Objectification of the sexual partner ceases, and a worshipful mindset takes its place. The tantra god and tantra goddess engage each other at the mind level and only proceed to the level of sacred sex.

Tantra meditation may lead to actual sex, but a physical encounter is by no means the only objective. Your tantra master will make it very clear that the most important objective of tantric meditation is complete mindfulness of the partner and of oneself. The sexual energy that exists between the intimate partners is examined and cherished at the mind level, and this itself can be far more exciting and fulfilling than even a full-body orgasm.

In practicing tantra meditation under a ⍰ualified tantric teacher, the students of tantra discover and explore the sacred aspects of their love for each other. Done correctly and consistently, it is a deeply transforming experience that cannot be matched by the mere joining of bodies at the physical level.

In the basic format of tantric meditation, the partners sit quietly in front of each other. They sit neither too near nor too far apart. They may be clothed or naked, and they may look upon each other or sit with their eyes closed. Either way, they are opening up a channel for tantra energy to flow freely between them.

If sex is to follow, the partners should decide on a period in which they will first engage in complete mindfulness and meditation before sex ensues. In this period, they will engage in tantra breathing and maintain a worshipful silence. Initially, their tantric master will guide their thoughts so that they do not stray from the desired focus.

When the partners have achieved a sufficient level of proficiency in this form of meditation, they are often able to achieve orgasms without so much as touching or looking at each other. No foreplay, erection or any kind of physical contact is required - it happens at the cosmic level.

If you are eager to explore the transformative powers of tantra meditation, you should seek out an experienced tantric teacher who can initiate and guide you into it. It is a grievous mistake to practice tantra without such expert guidance since amateur attempts can seriously contaminate any spiritual pursuit.

Tantric Journey

Tantric Journey is a holistic treatment program that incorporates Tantric and Tao bodywork techniques alongside other recognized holistic modalities. The aim of the treatment is aiding people to gain release from negative trauma in order to overcome a range of physical, sexual and emotional difficulties including depression, sexual dysfunction, past trauma, low self-esteem, overcoming past abuse and increasing well-being.

Tantric Journey also provides training and education in the field of emotional release through bodywork and is committed to increasing awareness of work and techniques in this field.

Mal Weeraratne is the founder of Tantric Journey – School of Healing and Awakening and author of Emotional Detox through bodywork. Mal is a British pioneer of emotional release through bodywork, with over 20 years' experience, treating over 3500 clients from all walks of life from the UK, USA, Europe, and Asia.

Mal has developed Tantric Journey a healing and awakening technique based upon the ancient principles of Tantra and Tao in conjunction with groundbreaking

Western knowledge; to create a powerful and transformative form of therapy that is capable of releasing trauma at a cellular level within the body.

Chapter 9:Emotional and Cultural Consent

Tantric sex does require you to have consent, just like all forms of sex. But, it's a little different this time around. Consent in tantric sex is both emotional and cultural in aspects, and we'll highlight what each of these is, why they matter, and how to approach this.

Consent: Why It's Sexy

For most people, consent is something that should always be there, but it's something that not only allows for sexual situations to be a mutually-beneficial activity, but it's also the difference in many cases between sex and of course, rape and abuse.

Consent is something that you should always work towards having. Most people don't understand the impact nonconsensual activities are on someone, whether it be sex or otherwise, and consent allows for you to subject yourself to this, so you're happier and healthier.

But consent isn't just in a physical consent. The whole "I'm okay with you touching me there" is impactful, but it's more than just a physical action.

Also, it's an emotional, mental, and cultural type of agreement.

Physical consent is usually given in most relationships. You say it's okay to have sex, and then you do it. But tantric sex requires emotional and cultural consent, and both of these are something that usually most sex doesn't have. Sex can be emotional, but usually, you don't need heavy emotional consent when you're having sex. But, with tantra, it is a very emotional activity, and you need to understand that, in order to have a successful tantra experience, you must give the consent to experience the emotions of yourself and other people.

What Is Emotional Consent

Emotional consent is where you consent to the emotions that someone else either gives to you, or you provide.

Have you ever talked to someone where, at first, it's just you talking about your problem, but your friend suddenly jumps forward, giving unsolicited advice on how to handle the situation? Have you ever done this? Oftentimes, emotional consent is just as important as physical consent. It isn't good to be on either side of those types of interactions, and for most people, jumping into that oftentimes means that your conversations will be disappointing, and it can oftentimes be very frustrating to deal with.

The problem is that we live in a world that's messy, and you need to understand that you have to build deeper connections with other people that you come into contact with. But the thing is, you need to give the okay to experience those types of emotions. To do otherwise allows you to build trust with the other person, and it leaves you both a place to share your thoughts.

Talking to others is tiring. Emotional labor is something that most of us don't sign up for, and emotional consent is very important because it honors the ability to give the other person the perspective that you have, and also, so that they're not being bombarded with these emotions and instead, you both set healthy, happy boundaries with others.

Emotional consent is as simple as you're both okay with feeling the effects of it, and also how you can benefit from this as well.

Emotional consent is more than just "I'm willing to listen to your problems," though. Lots of times, emotional consent in tantra is allowing yourself to be exposed to some of the harsher realities of the world.

When you experience tantra, you go through a lot of emotions, and oftentimes, you both have to be on the same page. Breathing together, looking at one another, experiencing the flow of one another's energies can be tough, especially after a long day. That's why, if you practice tantric sex, it's important to do this when you're not hung up on the distractions of life, and instead, you're able to easily understand and utilize the information that you learn about your partner.

It's a very spiritual activity, and you need to consent to get into those kinds of emotions. Sometimes, when you do this too, you tackle traumatic points.

Tackling Trauma and Emotional Consent

The emotions you experience during tantric sex aren't just the emotions of yourself and the other person. Tantric sex is done to free yourself from the bindings of other people, and oftentimes, what people don't realize is that with tantric sex, it can be a very stimulating process for both parties.

Tantric sex involves looking at the traumatic associations with sex too. For many of us, we don't spend time enjoying the moment and the emotions associated with this. But, with tantric sex, we can overcome the problems of the past, and from there, face the future. However, you need to understand that it is an emotionally-stimulating thing, and it can be good for you, but also very heavy. Understand that you're also opening yourself up to the trauma and problems that your partner faces too, which is why many people don't realize the full power of tantric sex. For most of us, tantric sex helps us understand our own personal wellness and the ability to explore the unknown.

Consenting to this is important. Consent is something that you need to have emotionally and sexually during tantric sex. You need to understand that you must freely give consent, are giving informed consent, are enthusiastic abut I and you communicate with the other person what's going on.

Communicating, especially during the more traumatic elements, might be good for you. It lets you explore these desires and these feelings in a healthy way. Remember, you're also looking at sexual boundaries, eliminating them, and being free, which will, in turn, help you with improving your own wellness and happiness. Consent is really good not just for looking at the emotional aspects of I, but also to handle trauma related to this subject, which is more common than you think.

Consent as a Culture

Tantric sex encourages you to consent to everything that you do fully. That's the culture of it. When you engage in tantra, the goal of it is liberation, and you need to agree to the idea that, with tantra, you're going to experience new things related to it, and it can be a big thing for most people.

You need to understand that you should speak up for yourself and your own personal feelings. You shouldn't just blindly follow what the doctrines teach you, or if you're doing it with someone know knows tantra, also work to form your own conclusions as well. You should stay within your comfort zones in relation to tantra in order to minimize any changes of later regrets.

Always state your boundaries during tantric sex. If you like the massaging feeling of being touched in some areas, but not in other areas, you should always make sure you let the person know that you're with.

You should understand as well that you should never do group coercion either. Never just feel like you need to do something because it's said. Some people are definitely better by discussing things, and the culture of tantra encourages you to discuss this with the other person, so both of you are on the same page, and are honest with one another.

When doing tantra, always make sure to have honest feedback in place when doing this. If there are some things that you didn't like, let your partner know, and some things that you do like, again, let them know as well. You should always practice mutual consent with your partner, and make sure that you're both on the same page.

And as always, understand that tantra is a very personal thing. You don't need to scream to everyone about what happened during your five-hour tantric sex experience. That's something that should only be discussed between both of you, and not something that you should just keep out in the open. Keep the confidentiality of it in place, because it'll help with improving the sexual experience, and the wellness you share as well.

Boundaries Still Matter in Tantra

Finally, remember your boundaries in tantric sex is still a big thing here. That's because, even though tantric sex involves going with the flow and doing things that stimulate your mind along with the body, you have to understand that there are still some boundaries that you shouldn't cross.

If that ever gets violated, that's not okay. That's assault, and that's something that you should never have happens. Instead, be honest with your partner, and you should also make sure that boundaries are discussed in a way that's fitting for everyone, and in a way that's safe.

As always, just like with any other type of sexual experience, it's very important you keep your consent in place, and you try to work on being consensual, and also willing to work together. You should try to as well, make sure that you understand the value of consent, and what happens when you consent with your partner. Discuss this early on, but always make sure that you do have these worked out, both physically and emotionally, and the type of cultural consent you'll have.

Cultural consent can be something as simple as tying a ritualistic experience with it or wearing similar clothing to signify it. Always talk with your partner before you begin with this, and make sure you're both on the same page regarding it, because that alone will help improve your experience.

Chapter 10: Tantric Sex Tips

The principle motivation behind Tantra is to assist you with accomplishing splendid climaxes that you have been precluded because from securing your standard sexual practices. Notwithstanding, this doesn't imply that Tantra ought to be dealt with daintily. Consider Tantra an erotic exercise. Tantric sex is viewed as more charming than going through hours together at the rec center. Yet, the measure of physical effort that your body encounters can be contrasted with that you may be understanding while at the same time playing out any overwhelming activities.

Additionally, there are various degrees of Tantric sex. Essentially bouncing into Tantra with no experience or primer practice may improve your sexual coexistence, yet it is so much better when you participate in some type of pre-sex warm-up practice that will help in setting the mindset and working up some expectation concerning what is yet to come. There are a few manners by which you can heat up. However, perhaps the most ideal way that could be available is to give your partner a back rub and have your partner give you one also. This will extricate up your muscles, which is significant in light of the fact that solid muscles can hinder a full-body climax.

The back rub that you are providing for setting up your darling for tantric sex has some particular standards that are joined to it, alongside a system that is intended to uplift the sexual affectability and make the body progressively open to assist sexual incitement. Additionally, this back rub can be combined with a procedure that can be used on a lady to cause her to accomplish a climax. This will contribute extraordinarily to the nature of tantric sex in light of the fact that accepting one climax makes an individual patient for the following one, and this furnishes you with the fundamental open door o coax your partner and draw out the sex.

The Use of Oil

The main thing that you need before you can give your sweetheart a pre-sex knead is oil. Oil is an incredible instrument that can be used if you need your back rub to be increasingly compelling. It helps in extricating the skin up and giving grease to your hands. If your hands can slide and coast easily over your darling's body all the more adequately, then it will likewise help in making the back rub increasingly sexy and causes in paving the way to the real sex!

The best oil that you can use in a pre-sex rub is grape seed oil. This is because grape seed oil has a minimal number of individuals that are oversensitive to it, and can be incredible for your skin. In this manner, by giving your sweetheart a grape seed oil rub, you will be helping him, or she gets milder skin too, and isn't this a fantastic special reward? You can generally include a couple of drops of your preferred scented or basic oil to make the experience far and away superior. Distinctive fundamental oils can be used, relying on the specific explanation behind which it is being used. For example, lavender can be used for unwinding and alleviating muscles; rose can be used for giving an increasingly erotic feel to the back rub.

If grape seed oil isn't accessible, go for whatever other oil that has been made with the end goal of back rubs.

The Technique

The primary thing that you should do is clearly begin spreading the oil over your sweetheart's body. Ensure that the oil is conveyed uniformly everywhere throughout the body, and remember that too little oil won't give sufficient oil and result in teasing. In any case, using an excess of would simply wind up getting chaotic, and this can be irritating. Attempt to locate the fair compromise! While you are spreading the oil over your partner's body, you will find that the skin ingests the oil rapidly. Thus, you should keep habitually spreading more oil over their body, if the grease quits being adequate.

When the oil has been spread over your partner's body, the back rub can appropriately start. At first, it would be a smart thought to begin with the essential pressure of the entirety of the significant muscles. The muscle you ought to go for while applying wide and vague pressure are the thigh muscles since this zone is normally under the most strain for the duration of the day.

When the muscles have been relaxed up in your partner's legs, you can move their back, the second-most tense region of the normal body. Simply apply pressure with your straightened palm, and make sure to speak with your partner as much as you can about what feels better and what is excruciating.

Attempt gently slapping territories that you feel are as of now free to invigorate blood courses in these zones. Recollect not to slap so hard that it harms except if your partner needs you to obviously!

When you have finished this back rub and released up the significant muscle gatherings, the time has come to start centered pressure with the tips of your fingers and your clench hands. There are explicit territories that you ought to focus on centered pressure, and these zones are determined in the following segment.

Territories to Target

Bosoms: The bosoms are one specific territory of the human life systems that will work in a general draw in a great deal of consideration, and it so occurs that they are additionally an astounding wellspring of sexual incitement for some individuals. They likewise will, in general, have exceptionally thought purposes of strain that, when discharged, wind up, causing the individual to feel fantastically loose and quiet.

Along these lines, bosoms are clearly going to be one of the most significant zones of the body that you should target. Purposes of pressure here are most likely going to be on the lower half of the bosoms. It is significant that you search, attempting to discover the zone where the pressure exists.

This little wad of strain can be discovered right beneath the areola, and your partner may likely shout out when you hit this specific spot. In any case, don't confound this torment and stop the back rub. This torment is entirely charming, with numerous individuals contrasting it with the inclination once gets while scratching a tingle.

Something imperative to note while performing such a back rub is the source of these little wads of strain that are available in the body. They are not just strong pressure. Their root is more mystical than physical in nature.

You are as of now acquainted with the different chakras present in the body. In any case, you most likely don't know that these chakras are the significant stops in an immense system of energy that is streaming inside your body, vortices through which energy continually streams. However, there are certain circumstances where the progression of energy can get disturbed.

This typically occurs because of a less than stellar eating routine or a physical issue in a previous existence that may residually affect your body right now. Therefore, when you apply profound strain to these points, the energy begins to get discharged, consequently expelling the impediment that was formerly hindering the progression of energy in your body.

Discharging energy is agonizing and yet very charming in light of the fact that the progression of energy gives essentialness and expanded sexual affectability to your body. This implies when you knead these points, your partner is going to feel an extraordinary tingling vibe that will regress into a stimulating sensation as the blockage is expelled from the energy pathways in the body.

An ideal manner by which you can apply strain to this specific point is by pushing down using the tips of your fingers. Start by applying pressure and moving your hands in a round movement. This will discharge the energy blockage in a mellow and proficient manner. The round movement extricates up stuck energy and afterward permits your hand to move away to an alternate piece of the blockage, permitting the relaxed up energy to stream into the energy pathway without being impeded by the pressure of your fingers.

You can likewise apply serious strain to this point. This is exceptionally valuable since it will discharge energy from the blockage in a very serious way, and this will wind up opening your partner up for extraordinary sexual incitement.

Butt: This is another zone of the body that a great many people are stirred by. For reasons unknown, the butt is similarly as inclined to blockages in energy as bosoms seem to be, most likely in view of the extraordinary sum strain they experience when the individuals they are appended to spend by far most of their day sitting in an office. With the measure of sitting that we do, it is no big surprise that the pathways of energy in our derrieres wind up getting sponsored up.

The significant thing here is to feel your way around the territory. Blockages can happen in a few distinct pieces of the butt, so you should look around a little to discover where precisely the blockage has happened. An odd little fortuitous event is that the energy blockage is likely going to happen in a similar spot on the two cheeks, so if you discover the spot on one cheek, basically begin squeezing a similar spot on the other cheek also.

Apply a similar round movement with the tips of your fingers that you used on your partner's bosom. These energy blockages may require some more pressure, notwithstanding, so if your partner can't feel anything when you are rubbing that person, simply having a go at using your thumb.

You may confront trouble finding the pressure point right now the body, particularly if your partner has been skilled with a breathtaking posterior. This is because the energy pathways are covered underneath a great deal of substance. Bosoms once in a while ever posture such an issue, regardless of whether the bosoms being referred to are huge.

This is because the pressure points situated in bosoms are not as profound as the ones in the rear. Henceforth, if you are confronting troublesome finding your partner's pressure point, use your thumb, and it will work. If your thumb is as yet not adequate, have a go at using something inflexible like a pen to apply pressure, simply ensure you use the backside of the pen and not the pointy end!

Using such a device will assist you with providing unimaginably engaged pressure onto the energy blockage, encouraging a speedy scattering of energy and in the process most likely turning your partner on a lot.

Internal thighs: Finding the blockage in energy right now, your body may end up being significantly more troublesome than discovering it on different pieces of the body. This is the reason a cursory back rub of the thighs is important before you start to test for pressure points.

The muscle rub is useful because it will expel many interruptions from that general region. A great deal of the time, you may be examining for the pressure point and would as far as anyone knows think that its rapidly, just to find that it was simply fundamental muscle torment and not the agony that originates from a blocked energy pathway.

However, if you have loosened up the muscles in your partner's thighs, the procedure ought to be significantly simpler. One great tip that you ought to follow is to search for the pressure point in the upper internal thigh, which implies the territory of your thigh that is legitimately beneath your partner's groin.

Attempt to crush this zone for the most part to locate a general area of the pressure point, and afterward slender it somewhere near using the tips of your fingers. When you discover the pressure point, begin applying a similar roundabout pressure that you used to both the past body parts.

Be careful while applying strain to the internal thighs. The pressure point here is significantly more sensitive than the pressure points in the butt or even the bosoms. Delicate pressure will take care of business, and apply an excess of pressure will simply wind up, causing pointless agony that will likely power your partner out of the temperament.

If the round movement strategy ends up being unreasonably extraordinary for your partner, have a go at pushing your fingers ahead as you delicately knead the point. This will help by applying a lot of gentler pressure than the roundabout movement, and the way that it is significantly more arousing absolutely doesn't hurt either!

Lower back: This territory of the body is totally different from the three zones talked about beforehand, thus will handle in a way that is totally unique to how that the past body parts were handled

What makes the lower back so one of a kind is that it doesn't have a solitary purpose of energy blockage that you should concentrate on. Or maybe, your partner will have one of two potential energy blockage circumstances, every one of which has the particular system that you can use to handle it.

The principal circumstance would be that there are a few dozen separate purposes of energy blockage that are peppering over your whole lower back, being centered explicitly around the segment of your lower back legitimately before your butt alongside the region of your lower back that is straightforwardly along your spine.

The subsequent circumstance would be that the energy blockage would be spread out over the aggregate of your lower back, with the energy nexuses interconnecting to shape a system of blockages like the genuine system of energy pathways that your body has.

The subsequent circumstance is regularly found in ladies with huge bosoms and individuals who do a great deal of physical work. This is because such individuals will, in general, put a great deal of strain on their lower back, compelling the energy pathways to get blocked in light of the fact that these strenuous exercises would intrude on their flow.

By and large, the lower back is continually going to be an intense spot of energy blockage except if your partner gets customary back rubs, and the advantage of this is even the scarcest back rub right now significantly invigorate your partner and will bring about practically moment excitement whenever done right.

To discover which of the two-energy blockage circumstances your partner is experiencing, you will need to test a considerable amount. Use your fingers to see where the energy blockages are. If there are spaces between the points where your partner feels torment, this implies the energy blockages that your partner is experiencing are isolated from one another.

Nonetheless, if every last bit of your partner's spinal pains when you rub it in that extraordinary bothersome, tickly way, then your partner's energy blockage circumstance is of the subsequent kind.

The principal circumstance is significantly harder to handle than the subsequent circumstance. Since the energy blockages are not associated, you will need to handle every one independently as opposed to all simultaneously. This is because endeavoring to knead a few points without a moment's delay could bring about terrible agony for your partner.

In any case, settling this energy blockage circumstance isn't that troublesome once you get its hang. Just press each pressure point and discharge the blockage by moving your hands in the roundabout movement that you will be recognizable to at this point. You will find that once you deal with one blockage, the ones around it will start to get more fragile consequently.

This implies concentrating on a few significant spots will permit you to scatter the energy blockages and have the energy pathways streaming openly in the blink of an eye.

The subsequent circumstance, in any case, requires an altogether different methodology. The main thing you should think about this methodology is that it includes positively no nuance. The energy blockage is serious and will hinder your partner's climax, and since the blockage is across the board and interconnected, the best thing that you can do is attempt to handle at quite a bit of it simultaneously as you can.

Warm up your partner's lower back by using your thumbs to slide the energy blockages into getting somewhat more fragile. Following a moment or two of this, you should start using your clench hands. Ply your partner's lower back as though it was the batter. This may appear to be clever, however, if you ply your partner's lower back precisely how you would massage mixture, with the snappy developments and not remaining in a similar spot for a really long time, your partner will before long be loose to such an extent that they'd feel as if they are drifting endlessly.

The subsequent circumstance, albeit in fact increasingly serious, is significantly simpler to disperse than the primary circumstance. Simply ensure that you don't wind up harming your partner by applying an excessive amount of pressure. Keep in mind, and correspondence is fundamental if you need to ensure that the back rub experience is as pleasant as could be allowed.

You will find that no other zone will give as a lot of sexual incitement as the lower back as it is being rubbed. This is because the energy that is being discharged is making them much progressively touchy to sexual improvements. Giving your partner a full body climax will turn into significantly simpler after you have rubbed her back to the furthest reaches conceivable.

Chapter 11: Spiritual Phase of Sexual Energy

The Ecstasy of Tantra and Tao

Many people yearn for a different experience of sexuality, an enlightened union of sex and spirit with one's lover.

The Eastern philosophies of Tantra and Tao embody this kind of mind/body/spiritual approach toward sexuality. These disciplines seek to elevate the art of lovemaking, transforming intimacy into a form of worship, a journey of sacred self-discovery and an opportunity to transcend ordinary personal boundaries.

These belief systems evolved thousands of years ago geographically rooted in Tibet, China and India. Elaborate ancient texts describe lovemaking in detail with the essence of sexuality steeped in religious symbolism.

Tantra

Tantra is a philosophy and a belief system enacted through a variety of rituals, many dealing with activities of daily life such as eating, bathing and meditating. Other rituals worship the sanctity of the body including purifying the body for prayer; preparing the body for sexual activity, and a host of activities regarding specific sexual and spiritual acts.

Tantra reveres sexuality, viewing the act of sex as a form of divine worship, an intimate form of communication with a higher power.

Tantra is still evolving when it comes to religion, symbolism and the path to the divine. What we all do know and feel, however, is that Tantra is becoming synonymous with the concept of "spiritual sex" or "sacred sexuality.

The principle, once again, is that sex should not be regarded as merely a pleasurable sensations but a sacred act of "worship" if you will, one that could even lead to a more sublime state of mind or spiritual traveling experience.

The Expanded Orgasm: This refers to an experience that seeks to heighten the orgasm of the male or female, so that it goes well beyond the norm. Some people describe it as a "full body orgasm" rather than a genital orgasm. Allegedly, some people (including Patricia Taylor, PhD) have documented cases of individuals orgasming for an hour or even hours upon adequate stimulation. Here we see the "bliss" of Tantra and other eastern disciplines; the orgasm is oftentimes related to the entrance of divine thought and feeling.

Orgasm Control: The second part of sex magic is that of putting off orgasm, or orgasm control. This involves a person (male or female) achieving a high level of sexual arousal for a long period of time, but refraining from ejaculation or orgasm. This is due not only to heighten the orgasm later on but also to help the other partner (usually female) reach orgasm at the same time or within a short time. This is the disciplinary action, the mental exercises, that Tantra stresses so that lovers can get their minds out of the typical genital response cycle, and instead think "bigger."

Tantra has become synonymous with the concept of "spiritual sex" or "sacred sexuality. The principle, once again, is that sex should not be regarded as merely a pleasurable sensations but a sacred act of "worship" if you will, one that could even lead to a more sublime state of mind or spiritual traveling experience.

The Expanded Orgasm: This refers to an experience that seeks to heighten the orgasm of the male or female, so that it goes well beyond the norm. Some people describe it as a "full-body orgasm" rather than a genital orgasm. Allegedly, some people (including Patricia Taylor, Ph.D.) have documented cases of individuals orgasming for an hour or even hours upon adequate stimulation. Here we see the "bliss" of Tantra and other eastern disciplines, the orgasm is oftentimes related to the entrance of divine thought and feeling.

Orgasm Control: The second part of sex magic is that of putting off orgasm, or orgasm control. This involves a person (male or female) achieving a high level of sexual arousal for a long period of time, but refraining from ejaculation or orgasm. This is due not only to heighten the orgasm later on but also to help the other partner (usually female) reach orgasm at the same time or within a short time. This is the disciplinary action, the mental exercises, that Tantra stresses so that lovers can get their minds out of the typical genital response cycle, and instead think "bigger."

The sexual rituals culminates in a sublime experience of infinite awareness for both lovers. Tantric texts specify that sex has three distinct and separate purposes- procreation, pleasure, and liberation. Lovers seeking enlightenment may avoid frictional and opt for a static embrace with deep eye gazing.

The sexual act balances energies coursing in the channels of both partners. When the Kundalini force, a psycho-spiritual energy, the energy of the consciousness, is awakened is spirals upwards in the body. This kindles sexual energy which is harnessed for union with the spiritual. Both partners dissolve into a state of cosmic consciousness.

One of the basic tenets of Tantric teachings is a man riding the wave of sexual arousal without ejaculating. He is able to experience extreme pleasure through meditation and deep breathing. With practice a man can learn the art of arousal without ejaculation allowing himself and his partner prolonged time for mutual exploration.

In this heightened state of arousal, lovers can transcend the physical act of sex characterized by rubbing and friction, and climb toward a spiritual exchange of souls. This is often called The Soul Orgasm.

Taoism

The fundamental teachings of Taoism are based on the teachings of its founder Lao Tzu who believed that energy flows throughout all life.

In ancient China, Taoist masters were respected for their specialized knowledge of human sexuality. Sex was not merely a physical act, but a way of attaining a long and healthy life. Sexual energy was associated with vibrant health, sharp senses, an intelligent mind, and the balancing of masculine and feminine energies, the yin/yang

Taoists believe that when lovemaking occurs partners "join energy" and thus experience a wealth of health and spiritual benefits. Sex involved universal energy (qi) and a balancing force (jing).

Preserving the precious jing was of utmost importance for a man to maintain good mental and physical health.

The most potent form of jing was semen. Therefore, the more a man ejaculated, the more likely he would deplete his jing, robbing himself of essential nutrients.

Above all, Taoists believed that ejaculation should be withheld to allow the elements in the ejaculate to circulate throughout the body like a highly potent vitamin pack.

Integrating Sexuality and Spirituality

Take a look at the world around us, and it becomes readily apparent that we are living in a time of simultaneous convergence and deconstruction. As there is a resurging interest in spiritual practices in many circles, there is also a breakdown in the patriarchal, hierarchical church structures. The specter of clergy sexual abuse intermingles with a worldview promulgated by the church about the nature of relationships and sexuality that no longer has meaning for people today - men and women, young and even middle-aged. The gender roles we were raised with have broken down and blurred. The image of nuclear family as mom, dad and 2.4 children has been superseded by a far greater spectrum of family possibilities. Bisexuality, androgyny, gender fluidity and polyamory are more and more common, especially among the twenty something generation.

Erotic energy is far more than sexual energy. It is life energy. As our culture has evolved splits between mind and body, head and heart, heart and pelvis and sexuality and spirituality, we have forgotten what it means to be fully alive.

"Erotic energy is not just about having sex," continues Suzanne Blackburn, whose participation in sexuality and spirituality work has catapulted her personal and spiritual growth. "It is about living." As we have become disconnected from our bodies, hearts, souls, spirits, one another and the divine, we have lost touch with many of the most beautiful pleasures and experiences possible in being human. So many people today are searching for meaning and purpose, most often expressed through job dissatisfaction, addictions and broken or troubled relationships. The rise of industrialization, urbanization, the nation-state, global dislocations, war and poverty all contribute to the sex-spirit split for us both individually and collectively.

"Because our culture has repressed sexuality so much, it is repressing everything," acknowledges Blackburn. "People who have repressed sexuality have also repressed other areas of their lives. If you are not joyful about your sexuality, it is hard to be joyful about watching a sunset or watching kittens play. Hopefully, by breathing life into one, you breathe life into all of it. It's like giving birth. When the baby comes out of the birth canal and takes a breath, the baby pinks up. When we open up, breathe deeply, have fun, when we dance, we pink up." This backdrop provides fertile soil for an emerging movement working to integrate sexuality and spirituality.

Living in the Midst of a Paradigm Shift

Just as Western civilization went through a period of major cultural upheaval 2000 to 3000 years ago, we are undergoing a period of major cultural turnover and paradigm shift now. "The institutional churches are losing their credibility in dealing with sexuality and spirituality. They are losing their authority," continues Francouer. Francouer is well versed in the changing paradigm worldwide. The International Encyclopedia of Sexuality is written by 300 experts in 60 countries on 6 continents. The encyclopedia includes in depth reports of all aspects of sexuality. Each country has a section on religious and ethnic influences. Having collected information from many cultures all over the world, "it becomes very clear the spiritual traditions are undergoing major revolutions in their patterns of thinking. People in many cultures worldwide are thinking now not in terms of marital and procreational values, but in terms of individual self-enrichment and fulfillment. The spiritual is a very important part of the new perspective."

Significant leadership in the sexuality and spirituality is coming from women. Francouer acknowledges, "As women in developing nations are exposed to Western concepts and experiences of human sexuality, they are linking their religious traditions with the visions of Western sexuality. As women become more empowered in third world nations, they are gaining more control over their bodies and sexuality, turning more to their spiritual heritage."

"When the human psyche reaches the point of convergence and breakthrough into a new level of consciousness," reflects Francouer, "diversity is the first thing that happens. The energy spreads out and explores all kinds of possibilities. There is no one ideal paradigm nor five ideal paradigms. All the models we have had in the past have real difficulties being applied in today's world. So people are creating their own models and patterns."

The new paradigms created need to include and consider the collective as well as the individual.

A Quiet Movement and Its Roots

The emergence of the sexuality and spirituality movement is very quiet. For one, the subjects of sexuality and spirituality are each daunting. Many people are frightened at the thought of delving more deeply into either one. Too, Ani Colt, publisher of Spirituality and Sexuality magazine and founder of the Sexuality and Spirituality Union Network (SUNetwork) points out, "One of the things that energized a lot of movements was the common experience of feeling oppressed. A sense of oppression contributed to the emergence of blacks, women and homosexuals. But the oppression of our sexuality is not even recognized because sex is always in front of us. It's in ads, on TV, in the movies. It is much more subtle oppression. As a result, it hasn't given us that organizing energy that has created the feminist movement, the civil rights movement and the gay, lesbian, bisexual and trans gendered community."

Sex educator, sex coach and author Loraine Hutchins adds, "Erotophobia/sex-negativity is hard to battle because it is all pervasive and systemic. It doesn't affect any one group at the expense of another like racism. However, erotophobia, like racism, really hurts everyone and diminishes us all. I think sex-negativity is a function of heterosexism, a system of oppression created by patriarchy, involving male supremacy and mandatory heterosexuality. This oppressive system hurts men as well as women. The parallel is in looking at how whites are made less by racism, in contrast to non-whites. The hurts are different and need different remedies."

"Organized religion is of little help in the sexuality-spirituality field," Shalom Mountain Retreat Center founder Gerry Jud acknowledges. "I make a big distinction between religion and spirituality. Religion is about controlling behavior. Spirituality is about development and liberation of consciousness - becoming consciousness itself. Sex permeates all of life. When people are intimate with each other, touch each other, look into each other's eyes, dance ecstatically with each other, the sexual component is out front. You cannot take an effective spiritual journey without taking into account that we are sexual beings."

The first nationwide survey on sexuality and spirituality was conducted by Gina Ogden, a sexuality therapist and author of Women Who Love Sex: An Inquiry into the Expanding Spirit of Women's Erotic Experiences. Oggen contends that the field of sexology itself has reinforced the split between sexuality and spirituality. While she was a visiting scholar at the Radcliffe Institute, she happened upon the earliest sex surveys - conducted by women MDs. "The first survey, a century ago, was filled with hand-written responses about sexuality and spirituality," notes Ogden. "But since the 1930's when male scientists took over the surveying of sexual behavior, sex research became focused on what was easy to count and measure - performance by way of intercourse, orgasms and spasms, the mechanical part." In her 25 years of experience as a clinician and workshop leader, Ogden found these mechanical features to be only a fraction of what women said was important.

"Almost 4000 women and men answered a survey with an outpouring of stories about sexuality and spirituality, about love and empathy and meaning and sex as a direct path to the divine. What is fascinating is that these stories echo the responses from those early surveys, as if they're filling in almost a hundred years of blanks, the mysterious black holes in the history of the sexuality and spirituality movement. Maybe the scientific arm of the present day movement begins with Celia Mosher, who conducted that first survey in 1892!"

Ogden continues, "There is brain research coming out now because with advanced technology like MRI's and PET scans we can really look at what is going on in the human brain over a period of time, like stop action. Researchers are finding that during sexual stimulation more than one center of the brain is lighting up. This demonstrates an organic basis for arguing that sexuality and spirituality are connected, that sexual response is multi-dimensional. This is in direct disagreement with all the sex research that focuses on performance, and the medical diagnostics that say if you can't perform to their standards, it's called dysfunction. There may be a political and social movement going on, but it's important to remember that the capacity for connecting sex and spirit is in us. It is in our cells and our brain structure. It is built in. It has taken us 3000 years to remember it, to rediscover it, to validate it."

A Wide Spectrum of Trainings and Practices

Many trainings, practices and methods have evolved to help people learn to work with sexual, spiritual, and life energies in their bodies, relationships and lives. These methods have been developed by visionaries who have built a community or network of people around them. There is some cross-fertilization between these communities, but more often the right hand doesn't even know there is a left hand yet, never mind what it is doing.

Existing practices and trainings approach integrating sexuality and spirituality from many different directions.

For example, the Human Awareness Institute approaches this work from an emotional and interpersonal direction, giving people skills for deeper intimacy and connection through its Love, Intimacy and Sexuality workshops. Tantric work, on the other hand, approaches the body and its energy field from a rootedness in spiritual philosophy. Sterling community work focuses on distinguishing the differences between male and female energy.

One of the common threads amongst the many approaches is the creation of a safe, sacred community circle. Joining together in holy ritual is a basic human need. We are starving for this kind of sacred circle. Trainings and workshops such as those profiled below provide help meet this need. I have selected a handful of significant programs in the sexuality and spirituality field, all of which have evolved over the past several decades. The purpose is to illustrate a range of what is available.

Chapter 12: Different Types of Sexual Play

There are many different types of sex. There's roleplaying, public, naughty, kinky, domination, and so on. And while some of them may seem downright odd to you or your partner, I would suggest trying a mild version of all of these in order to figure out what you two like in the bedroom together. Half the battle of having a great sex life is knowing what your partner likes, and the other half is knowing what you like.

Roleplaying

Everyone has fantasies, and if you're involved in a dedicated relationship but still find yourself thinking about getting it on with a hot police officer with some cuffs, don't be shy about asking your significant other to play out that fantasy. Roleplaying is a thrill for both people involved, and it gives partners that thrill of sleeping with other people without actually sleeping with others. It's a really great way to keep monogamy really hot. If you don't know where to begin with this type of sex, try some 'we don't know each other' sex. It gives you both the freedom to act as if you're someone else and take on a different personality, and allows you to do things you've always wanted to do but were afraid to ask for.

Exercise: Try going out to a restaurant with a bar attached and wait for your significant other to show up. Set it up ahead of time so the two of you can pretend not to know each other. You can also do this if you go to a park if you want it to be a little more secluded and private.

Splurge Sex

Have you ever noticed that when you go to a really nice place with your partner, the two of you seem to be amped up? Well, this is a phenomenon that occurs because the two of you are really excited about where you're at because it's different. So when you book that next vacation, splurge and go for a really nice room for at least one night so that the two of you can have a relaxing, adventurous day. You can even rent a hotel room in a city or town nearby that you know is really nice for one night, even if you're not going on vacation.

Public Sex

I'm not suggesting you get it on in the bathroom of a club, but if that's your thing, go for it. I am suggesting that if you go to the movies, sit in the back row, and guide his or her hand somewhere that's a little naughty. You don't have to do the entire deed in public, but get it started a little before you drive home to have some of the best sex of your life!

Beach Sex

There is a drink named after this act of sex on the beach, so it has to be amazing, right? You'll enjoy the crashing waves, the sun, and your hot partner with you. You don't have to limit yourself to lying down in the sand. The two of you could take a beach blanket, a lounge chair, or even have sex in the water.

Forbidden Sex

There's a book all about forbidden sex, and it's been a best seller for quite some time. Women and men both enjoy a little bit of kinkiness in the bedroom, so get out those handcuffs and figure out who's going to be the dominant one and who will be the submissive one for the evening. You don't have to live the BDSM lifestyle in order to try out a little taste of it.

Bathroom Sex

This is the most underrated room in the entire house for having sex. Seriously, it's a really great room! Try bending over the counter in doggie style position as your partner is behind you and watch his face as he takes you. Or sit on the counter so that he can see your backside at the same time that he's fondling your front. Men like a woman's sexy back and seeing the flow of her hair down her shoulders.

Makeup Sex

There are plenty of couples out there who will start a fight just because they know they're going to get makeup sex. I'm not kidding! Make up sex is charged with all that emotion that you just experienced, and it can be really steamy and hot. Women, don't resist the urge to have sex with a man after a fight. You're punishing yourself just as much as you're punishing him.

Lazy Sex

Sex does not have to be a marathon or a crazy ten-minute bout in the bedroom. The next time you're feeling lazy in the afternoon, or it's the morning and the weekend, take off all your clothes and snuggle up to your partner. Men and women's hormone levels are higher in the morning, and early afternoon, so it's a great time to have some really slow, connecting sex.

Loud Sex

All those four-letter words that you would never say in polite company are the ones that you want to use in the bedroom at least once during your relationship. Seriously, go all out and tell your partner exactly what you want him or her to do to you. Let them know how much you like it. The more explicit you are and the louder you are, the more excited they're guaranteed to be.

Random Sex

You know those times when you least expect your partner to jump your bones, and it happened? They were pretty exciting times, right? Well, return the favor to them! The next time you're walking through a secluded park, and it seems there isn't anyone else around, pull your partner to a private spot and get it on!

Chapter 13: Spicy Sex Positions

The Advantages of Using Different Sex Positions

When it comes to sex, changing the positions you use is the key to keeping it interesting and different. After a short time, a sexual routine can become boring and old, because you know what to expect at every turn and what to do next without thinking at all. Your brain, heart, and body do not need to be engaged like they are when you are doing something new and exciting that is really turning you on. When you are performing a sex position that you have never tried before, your entire body is engaged, thinking about what is next, feeling new sensations, looking to the other person to see if they are feeling pleasure as well. This is very different from performing a position you have done many times over. This is why changing your sex positions is beneficial; it engages every part of you.

Another advantage of using different sex positions is that they allow you to change and adjust according to what you are feeling and desiring on any given day. For some people, their desires may change quite often, and if they can recognize this, they will be able to choose the positions that feel right for them and meet their needs and desires every time they have sex.

Standing Suspended

This position requires strength from the man but can lead to very deep penetration if he is able to support his woman's weight enough. This position will be a workout for him, but a workout with a better ending than any workout he'll have in the gym!

The man stands facing the wall, and the woman stands in front of him, facing him. She puts her arms around his neck and jumps into his arms. He supports her weight by holding onto her butt cheeks while she has her arms and legs wrapped around him. He holds her up like this and lifts her higher to lower her onto his erect penis. Once inside, he can pin her against the wall for support so that he doesn't have to support her weight entirely and can use his hands to move her up and down on his hard member. If her back is supported by the wall, the man can also thrust into her using his hips if his arms get too tired. Because of the angle, the woman's legs are held at, her vagina and legs are open enough so that the man can penetrate her very deeply. This is one of the best positions if you want to attain very deep penetration. This increases the chances of the woman's G-spot being hit and will allow her to reach a G-spot orgasm that will drive her crazy!

The Rowing Boat

The rowing boat is another position that you may never have heard of. But, that will make for an exciting new sexual experience for you and your partner. This one begins with the man sitting on the floor or the bed with his knees bent and his legs spread. The woman will sit in exactly the same way, except she will be facing him. She will move her body toward him, and when they come as close as they can to one another, she will slide her knees underneath his knees, so that her legs are still bent, but underneath his. Her legs will then beholding his legs apart and open, and he will hold onto her legs to hold them open and bent. Then, he will slide his penis into her, and they can grind together for penetration to occur. This is an intimate position as you can both see each other's faces and are sitting with your legs spread right in front of each other. It is also intimate because it involves both people coming together with their bodies vulnerable and completely exposed, and their entirety open to their partner. This vulnerability will bring you both closer together, and this will lead to greater levels of intimacy and connection, especially since you will be able to see each other the entire time.

The Maid

This position is great for giving the woman blended or multiple orgasms of any sort, and this position is spicy because it incorporates a little bit of roleplay. This position is done on a ledge or a countertop, or even on the washing machine. Take this one to the kitchen for a nice change of scenery. The woman can even wear an apron with nothing else underneath to add a bit of a sexy roleplay element to this one if she wishes. The woman sits on the countertop with her legs spread, and her man stands in between her legs. She wraps her legs around him. He enters her from the front and will easily be able to hit her G-Spot in this position because of the angle of penetration. Having the woman sitting upright is a good way to ensure G-Spot contact. While he is hitting her G-Spot over and over, the pleasure will continue to build until she reaches an internal orgasm. If he continues to penetrate her in the exact same way at a steady rhythm, she will be able to keep feeling pleasure and keep having G-Spot orgasms over and over again. If she wants to try for a blended orgasm in this position, she can lean her upper body back against the cabinet and touch her clitoris as he is thrusting into her. This will lead to both a clitoral and G-Spot orgasm at the same time, and this means double the pleasure. He can continue to thrust into her even after this blended orgasm and she can then wrap her arms around his neck while he penetrates her without clitoral stimulation, and she will then have multiple vaginal orgasms after this. He will have to try hard to hold off his orgasm throughout all of this, as he will be very turned on by all of the pleasure his woman is feeling from his penis.

Make Your Sex Life Even Spicier: Anal Sex

Anal sex isn't something that everyone wishes to try, but if you are someone who is open to seeing what it's all about and why people like it. Anal sex can be enjoyed by everyone, any combination of genders and genitals. Anal sex is commonly associated with gay men, and straight men may be intimidated by the thought of being penetrated. Still, many men in heterosexual relationships enjoy being pegged by their female partners with a dildo or strap-on. This can be for couples with vaginas using a strap-on, couples with penises, or couples with a combination of both. Pleasure is universal, and so are these positions!

The Female Anus

The anus is a very sensitive area for women, contrary to the beliefs of some people. While it is well-known that men have sensitive anuses and can receive pleasure here, it is a less well-known fact that so can women. Women have very sensitive anal openings because there are many nerve endings present and a lot of surface area to work with. This means that when stimulated, a woman can feel a lot of pleasure here. Because this is an area that rarely receives a stimulation, when it does, it can be that much more enjoyable for a woman because she may not be used to the sensations.

The inside of the anus can give a woman lots of pleasure as well when stimulated. When a woman has her anus stimulated, it actually is only separated from the vagina by a thin layer, and similar to the clitoris and the G-Spot connection, she can actually orgasm from being anally stimulated because of the connection between her vagina and her anus. A woman can receive anal sex, and the penis making contact with her anal wall, especially the one toward the front of her body, can give her a very similar feeling to that of a vaginal orgasm.

The anus can also be stimulated with fingers, toys, or orally. Any of these ways can be enjoyable for the woman if she is open to receiving anal pleasure, as they will each give her a slightly different sensation. Think of how a warm tongue would feel vs. a smooth anal toy vs. the rough hands of the man she loves.

The Male Anus

The anus is a well-known erogenous area of the male body. Males can get intense pleasure and even orgasm from being anally penetrated. This is due to the prostate gland being positioned right sat the spot where whatever is doing the stimulating would make contact with the anal wall. Right on the other side of this wall is the prostate, which happens to be extremely sensitive and leads to intense pleasure when stimulated in the right way.

A man's anus can be stimulated on the outside only, where-like a woman's, it is very sensitive due to a great number of very sensitive nerve endings being located there. This can be done using a tongue, fingers, a vibrating toy, or anything really. Beginning with this will lead the anus to relax and become receptive to being penetrated. Then, a sex toy or fingers can be inserted, and that's when the prostate will get its turn. When they prostate it pressed on over and over in a rhythmic pattern, it will cause a man to feel intense pleasure and eventually to reach orgasm. This is similar to the G-Spot in a woman where it needs to be continuously stimulated in order to give her an orgasm eventually.

Anal sex for a man is not just reserved for gay couples. Many heterosexual couples practice pegging, which is anal sex from a woman to a man using a sex toy. We will revisit this later, but this point is to say that the pleasure potential of a man's anus is not only reserved for gay couples and should be fully explored by any man or heterosexual couple wanting to unlock the full pleasure that a man's body is capable of.

Conclusion

Tantra is the ultimate love affair with yourself and all of your existence. In the process of igniting your internal flame, you come to experience all ordinary moments as extraordinary experiences. Immersed in the experience, you realize that you are the divine, there is nothing else to need or want, but that moment. The Tantra is thus a great movement for the uplift of human existence, for the recovery of the whole of man to god. All life is sought to be spiritualized and given high value as a field and means for the manifestation of the divine. Not only in its aim but in its method too. The Tantra seeks to extend the claim of the spirit on all the members of the society.

The special characteristic features of Tantras are that they are extremely liberal and open to all castes and both sexes without any restrictions. This catholicity of the Tantric religion stood on the one hand against the Vedic practices and the metaphysical philosophy of the Upanishads and on the other, controlled the general mass by the force of energy of its magical appeal. In general, it is an attempt to point out that the tantric practices serve the function of helping practitioners to achieve a state of pure concentration.

Tantra art is based on rituals, which includes Yoga, offerings. Meditation and sexual intercourse. The most important concept found in the Tantras is the necessity of unifying apparent opposites in order to attain enlightenment. These opposites are usually represented as male energy (Shiva) and female energy (Shakti) or as the individual (Purusha) and nature {Prakriti). This the e⍰uality, or complementarily, of male and female, is a foremost aspect of tantric practice, as the union of both is required in order to achieve the highest understanding.

Tantra lies at the nexus of a series of conflicting extremes—the archaic past and the modern age of darkness; sexual liberation and sexual depravity; political freedom and political violence—each of which is seized upon in different historical moments. Perhaps most importantly, we have found that the image of Tantra has progressively shifted from a tradition associated with secrecy, danger, and occult power to one associated primarily with sexual liberation and physical pleasure.

Tantra is not something meant to be read about in books. What the text consists of are prescriptions for action including mental action which are the whole purpose of the texts. If you don't do what your Tantras describe, then you will never get the point.

Made in the USA
Monee, IL
27 December 2021